Sciatica Pain Relief Without Back Surgery

*Simple Sciatica Exercises and Home Treatments from the
Back Pain and Sciatica Clinic*

DR. JOHN FALKENROTH, D.C.

Back Pain and Sciatica Clinic

ISBN-13: 9798674539094

DEDICATION

This is dedicated to the countless number of people in this world who suffer from sciatica.

I have helped thousands of patients with sciatica for over 20 years now, and I hope that this material that I have put together will help sciatica sufferers like you get relief. I also want to help you avoid having your condition progress into something that is permanent and irreversible.

Since sciatica is a condition where people can't physically see what is wrong with you... you have no bruises, cuts, scrapes or wounds on your back or leg... it can be hard for others to empathize with your pain and suffering. All they see are the disabling functional effects of your sciatica.

Do not lose hope. I am here to help. My goal is to leave you feeling better than you did before you found this book.

Hopefully, after you read this book, you'll have a better understanding of your condition and you'll discover how you can relieve your sciatica, so that you can sit, stand, and sleep without sciatica, get your strength and flexibility back, and live a normal life free of sciatica.

I hope it is not too late for me to help you avoid back surgery.

Go to **www.repairmyback.com** and **www.sciaticaacademy.com** for more sciatica relief tips.

TABLE OF CONTENTS

Acknowledgments

1   What Is Sciatica?   1

2   How Sciatica Usually Starts and How It Gets Worse   5

3   Go Immediately to The Emergency Room If You Have This   11

4   Should You Get X-Rays or An MRI Of Your Spine?   17

5   The #1 Back Position You Must Avoid   23

6   Five More Common Activities You Should Avoid   27

7   How Smoking, Alcohol, and Excess Weight Affect Sciatica   33

8   The Proper Sitting and Standing Postures to Relieve Sciatica   37

9   Walk Forwards and Also Walk Backwards   43

10   Do You Have This Foot Problem Making Your Sciatica Worse?   51

11   Use This Formula to Determine How Much Water You Need   57

12   What Foods to Eat and What Supplements to Take   59

13   Making the Right Choice – Use Ice or Heat?   67

14   The One Rule You Must Follow When Doing Sciatica Exercises   71

15   The 6 Sciatica Exercises I Start My Sciatica Patients On   75

16   How to Keep Your Spine Aligned and Moving Properly   85

17   Can Massage Help Sciatica?   91

18   Painkillers, Muscle Relaxants, and Anti-Inflammatory Drugs   93

19	Should You Get Spinal Injections?	97
20	Is Sciatica Surgery Right for You?	101
21	Non-Surgical Spinal Decompression Therapy	113
22	How Aging Wreaks Havoc on Your Spine	117
23	What You Can Do to Slow Down the Aging of Your Spine	123

ACKNOWLEDGMENTS

Thank you to all my patients who have given me the privilege of trusting me with their spinal health. They have helped me gain the knowledge and the experience to help others like you who suffer from sciatica.

One of my greatest joys in life is helping people with back pain and sciatica by relieving their pain and suffering, improving their lives, and improving the lives of their family in the process.

Thank you also to all the wonderful teachers throughout my life who gave me a solid educational foundation and instilled in me the love of learning.

Finally, I want to thank my wonderful family – my wife Estrella and my three children James, Kevin, and Starlyn – for their unwavering love and support.

SPECIAL NOTE

1 WHAT IS SCIATICA?

Most commonly, sciatica is sharp or burning pain that goes from your lower back to the back of your legs. Symptoms can include pain in your low back, buttocks, back of your thigh, calf, or foot.

Instead of pain, you may experience numbness, tingling or weakness in your leg or foot. Sciatica is usually on one side only, but some people experience sciatica on both sides.

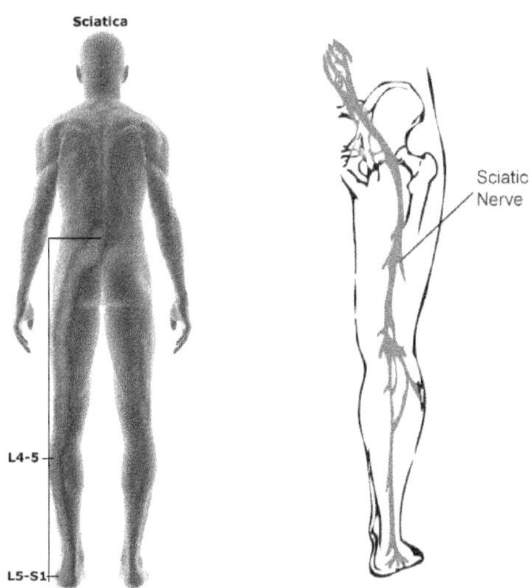

**The sciatic nerve travels from
the low back down to the feet.**

Why do you have sciatica? In short, because there is pressure on your sciatic nerve. Your sciatic nerve is made up of smaller nerve roots in your lower back - L4, L5, S1, S2, and S3. These nerve roots arise from your spine and join to form one large nerve called the sciatic nerve. Your sciatic nerve is about the size of your pinky.

If your sciatic nerve is compressed hard enough, muscle weakness can occur. You may notice difficulty standing on your toes. You may also develop a limp when you walk.

Time is of the essence. For some people, sciatica goes away on its own. However, without proper treatment, many people find that their sciatica gets worse.

If your sciatica does not get corrected fully, or soon enough, your sciatic pain may later be accompanied by or replaced by weakness of your affected leg muscles. This can cause a condition known as a "foot drop." Have you ever seen people dragging one foot when they walk? They might have uncorrected sciatica.

What can compress or irritate your sciatic nerve?

1. A lumbar herniated disc or disc bulge
2. Spondylolisthesis or a forward misalignment of a vertebra
3. Arthritic bone spurs on your spine where sciatic nerve roots exit
4. A tumor or cyst near or around your sciatic nerve or nerve roots

There are also other conditions that can cause "sciatica-like" symptoms. While these are technically not sciatica, the symptoms are the same. These conditions include:

1. An irritated or overly tight piriformis muscle
2. Referred pain from spinal facet joints
3. Diabetes or other metabolic conditions
4. Direct trauma to the buttocks or to the sciatic nerve

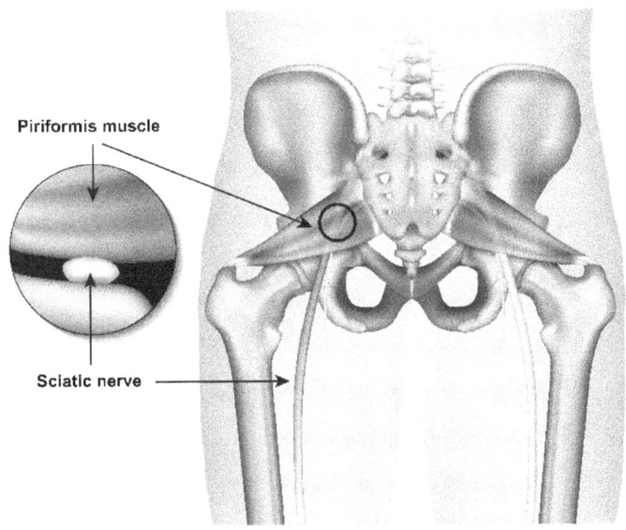

An inflamed, irritated, or overly tight piriformis muscle can compress and irritate the sciatic nerve on its path through the pelvis and down the leg

The sciatic nerve can get pinched by the piriformis muscle in the buttocks where the sciatic nerve passes through the pelvis. This has been commonly referred to as "wallet sciatica," since sitting on the wallet in the back pocket is often the cause.

When irritated, spinal facet joints can create referred pain. Usually, patients describe this referred pain as a "deep ache" inside the leg.

Metabolic diseases, such as diabetes, can damage nerves. If the sciatic nerve gets damaged, this is when people with metabolic diseases experience sciatica-like symptoms.

When you experience direct trauma to your buttocks, this can injure your sciatic nerve, and you can experience symptoms of sciatica. Direct trauma to your sciatic nerve can also lead to sciatica symptoms. For example, a needle can hit your sciatic nerve during an injection into your buttocks.

Dr. John Falkenroth, D.C.

2 HOW SCIATICA USUALLY STARTS AND HOW IT GETS WORSE

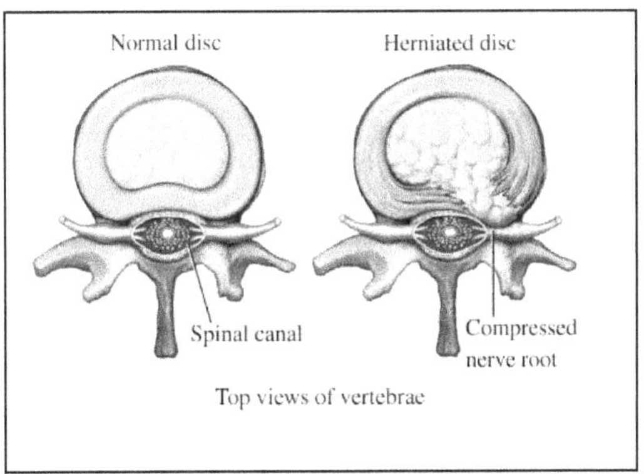

A herniated disc can pinch a nerve.

The most common cause of sciatica is a lumbar disc herniation or a severe lumbar disc bulge.

If we take things back one step further in figuring out the cause of sciatica, before the lumbar disc herniation or the disc bulge, sciatica probably started as abnormal movement or abnormal alignment of the bones in your lower back.

This abnormal alignment and movement can create uneven wear and tear on your spine, like the uneven wear and tear on your car tires when they're misaligned.

In the beginning, you may notice a clicking or a cracking sound when you move your back. This clicking or cracking sound with back movement is caused by the misaligned part of your spine rubbing abnormally against other parts of your spine.

You may also notice your low back muscles feeling STIFF - especially in the morning. You may find yourself massaging your back or trying to stretch your lower back throughout the day.

**Studies suggest that the longer
your spinal misalignments go uncorrected,
the GREATER your risk.**

If not treated properly, your condition will usually get worse. Unfortunately, uncorrected spinal misalignments will usually advance to more serious abnormal spinal conditions such as Spinal Arthritis, Bulged Discs, Herniated Discs, Degenerative Joint Disease or Spinal Stenosis. Any of these conditions can lead to sciatica.

Before developing sciatica, you might have felt a sharp pain, a dull ache or stiffness in your low back for days, months, or even years.

If your low back condition did not get treated properly, your low back pain may have progressed to sharp shooting pain, burning pain or numbness down your butt, back of your thigh, or back of your leg or foot. This condition is known as sciatica.

For some people, their sciatica comes and goes. If you pay close attention, you will notice that your leg pain, foot numbness or leg numbness usually gets worse with each episode or flare up.

In the beginning, your sciatica may be more of an annoyance versus being debilitating.

Unfortunately, your sciatica can quickly become serious and debilitating after doing even a MINOR activity such as sleeping the wrong way, sitting the wrong way, picking something up from the ground, pulling on something, or lifting something.

Many sciatica patients wake up one day with debilitating sciatica.

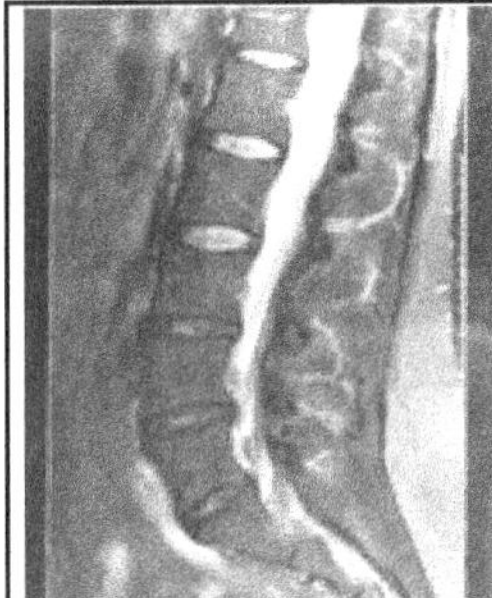

Notice the herniated discs in this lumbar spinal MRI. Bulged Discs and Herniated Discs like these can cause severe pinching of the delicate nerve roots that make up your sciatic nerve causing Sciatica.

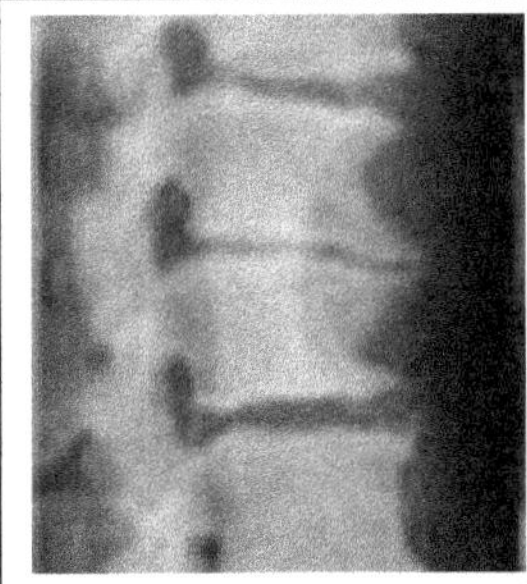

If you develop Spinal Arthritis or Degenerative Joint Disease in your low back, the bone spurs that you'll get from this condition may also pinch your sciatic nerve roots causing Sciatica.

As your condition gets worse, your sciatic nerve will degenerate or start to die. Because of this, you will lose function. Without proper sciatic nerve input, your thigh, leg and foot muscles on the side of your sciatica symptoms will get smaller and weaker.

In the beginning, it is harder to notice the muscle loss in your butt, thigh, leg, or foot. Have someone look at these areas and see if they notice muscle loss on the side where you feel your sciatica symptoms. In other words, have them look at you from behind and ask them to compare your left side and your right side. Is one side smaller than the other side?

If you lose muscle mass in your foot, you may notice that your shoe on the side of your sciatica will be looser than the other side. Because of your muscle imbalance, you may also notice that one of your hips is higher than the other hip, or that one of your legs is shorter than the other. This is called a functional short leg.

The imbalance between your right foot and left foot and your right leg and left leg can cause uneven wear patterns on your shoes.

Look at the bottom of the shoes that you normally wear. Do you notice uneven wear and tear patterns between your right shoe and your left shoe?

You may also notice being clumsier. For example, you may be tripping more often.

Besides losing muscle mass and strength, you will also most likely LOSE normal range of motion and flexibility in your lower back, hips, and possibly in your leg, ankle, and foot.

A lot of people can deal with the nagging sciatic nerve pain or sciatica numbness and tingling - especially when it comes and goes. But it's a lot harder for people to deal with the loss of function that comes later when their sciatica doesn't get fixed.

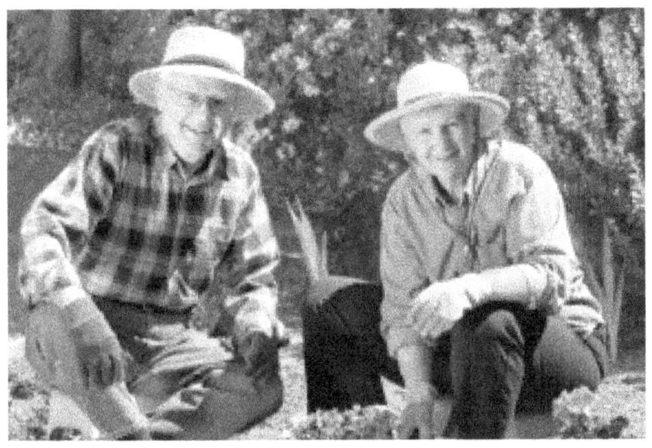

**If caught and treated early, most sciatica
can be fixed without much loss of function.**

However, untreated sciatica that progresses to the advanced degenerative stages almost always results in PERMANENT loss of function that will affect your activities of daily living - including your job, your hobbies, and your ability to take care of yourself and others.

For example, most of us take for granted being able to sit in the car and drive. But, if your sciatica gets worse, just the act of sitting in the car can be excruciatingly painful, making driving dangerous for you and for those around you.

The sooner you receive proper treatment for your sciatica, the better your chances of a FULL AND COMPLETE RECOVERY.

Sciatica is a complicated problem. It's best if you consult with someone who deals with sciatica patients all day long.

Otherwise, the wrong treatment can delay your recovery, or harm you, and can cost you thousands of dollars in unnecessary and ineffective treatments.

Dr. John Falkenroth, D.C.

3 GO IMMEDIATELY TO THE EMERGENCY ROOM IF YOU HAVE THIS

When sciatica does not get treated properly… or soon enough… or if your condition gets severe, you may develop Cauda Equina Syndrome.

What is Cauda Equina Syndrome?

It is a condition where you will notice numbness or loss of feeling in your lower body – your genitals, anus, inner thighs, heels, and feet. You may also experience sexual dysfunction.

You will also usually experience partial or complete loss of bowel and/or bladder control. Also, your legs will get weaker and weaker. Basically, you will feel like your lower body is getting paralyzed.

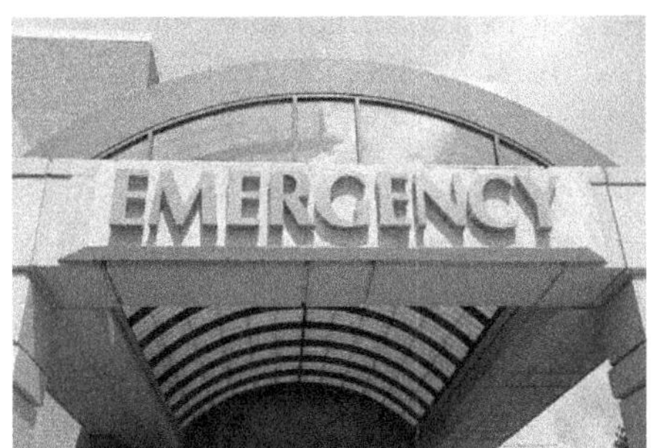

If you experience the scenario that I just described…
GO TO THE EMERGENCY ROOM RIGHT AWAY!!!

What exactly causes Cauda Equina Syndrome?

Let us cover a little bit of human anatomy here.

Your spinal cord ends around your upper to mid lumbar area. However, there are nerves and nerve roots that continue down below this area that look like a horse's tail… thus, the name Cauda Equina.

These nerves provide motor and sensory function to your lower limbs and to your pelvic organs such as your bladder and intestines.

When nerves in your Cauda Equina get compressed or injured, you get impaired or loss of motor and sensory function in the lower part of your body… you develop Cauda Equina Syndrome.

What causes this compression or injury to your Cauda Equina?

There are many different conditions that can cause Cauda Equina Syndrome. Here is a list of some:

- Massive herniated disc in the lumbar area
- Spinal tumor
- Spinal infection
- Lumbar spinal stenosis
- Spinal bleeding
- Complication of lumbar spine surgery
- Spinal anesthesia
- Pregnancy
- Spinal arteriovenous malformations (AVMs)
- Chronic spinal inflammatory conditions

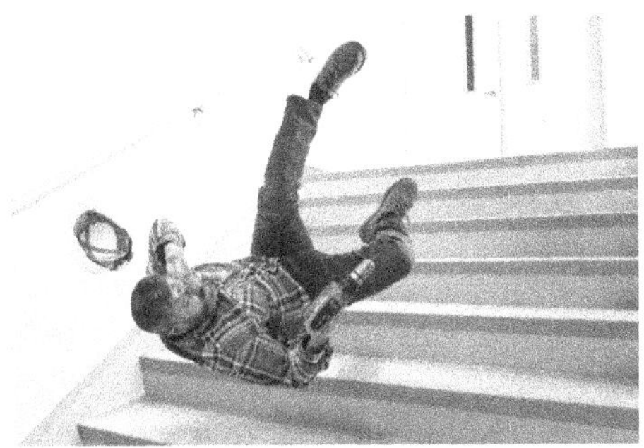

**Low back injuries from sports, falls, auto accidents,
knife wounds, or gun shots that cause fractures
or bleeding can also cause Cauda Equina Syndrome.**

Symptoms of your loss of <u>sensory function</u> can range from pins and needles to numbness or complete loss of sensation.

Symptoms of your loss of <u>motor function</u> can range from weakness to paralysis or complete loss of muscle function.

The severity of your loss of function will depend on the severity of the injury to your Cauda Equina nerves… and exactly which nerves are compressed or injured.

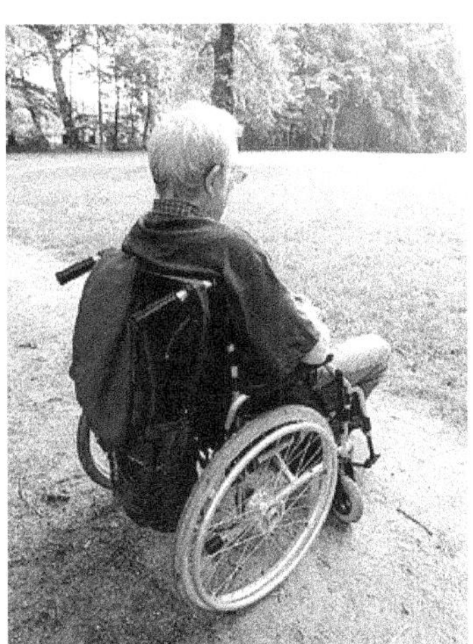

**Cauda Equina syndrome can happen
suddenly or gradually.**

The longer your condition remains untreated, the worse your prognosis.

Your treatment will depend on what is causing your condition.

If a tumor is causing your condition, you may need to get the tumor surgically removed and/or have radiation therapy or chemotherapy.

If an inflammatory condition like ankylosing spondylitis is causing your Cauda Equina Syndrome, then anti-inflammatory treatments will be used to relieve your symptoms.

Antibiotics may be used if your condition is caused by a bacterial infection.

Most Cauda Equina Syndrome is caused by something physical in your low back spine that needs to be removed such as a severe herniated disc, bone fragments, abnormal bone growth or blood.

At this point, emergency back surgery is your only treatment choice. Hopefully, your surgery will be successful and reverse your sensory and motor function loss.

Why do you need to go to the emergency room right away if you experience Cauda Equina Syndrome?

Cauda Equina Syndrome is considered a medical emergency requiring immediate surgery, because if not treated right away it can lead to bladder and bowel incontinence and permanent paralysis of your lower limbs.

Cauda Equina Syndrome can have a very negative impact on your work, relationships, and social life. You may lose your independence and your ability to take care of yourself and others.

Imagine having your lower limbs paralyzed and being incontinent. How would that affect your life and the lives of your friends and family?

You are also more likely to develop frequent urinary infections because you may not be able to fully empty your bladder.

Untreated Cauda Equina Syndrome can also lead to sexual dysfunction.

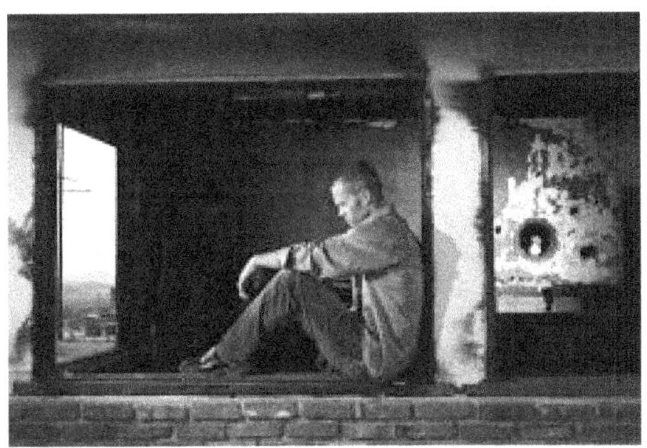

**The debilitating loss of function
of different parts of your body
can lead you to be depressed.**

Back surgery does not always immediately restore functional losses from Cauda Equina Syndrome. Sometimes, it can take years of healing, therapy, and hard work to bring back your lost bodily functions.

Unfortunately, a percentage of patients with Cauda Equina Syndrome never fully regain their bodily functions… even after back surgery.

Since a severe lumbar herniated disc is one of the main causes of Cauda Equina Syndrome, it's best if you take care of your spine… and if you experience lower back pain… that you get it treated right away and not let your condition get much worse.

4 SHOULD YOU GET
X-RAYS OR AN MRI OF YOUR SPINE?

Whether you need or should get X-rays or an MRI really depends on several factors. If you developed sciatica after an injury, and there is a possibility that you may have fractured your spine, get a spinal x-ray. CT scans may also be used to examine a spinal fracture more specifically.

If you are seriously considering back surgery to relieve your sciatica, you will need an MRI so that the surgeon can closely examine the current condition and structure of your spine before your surgery.

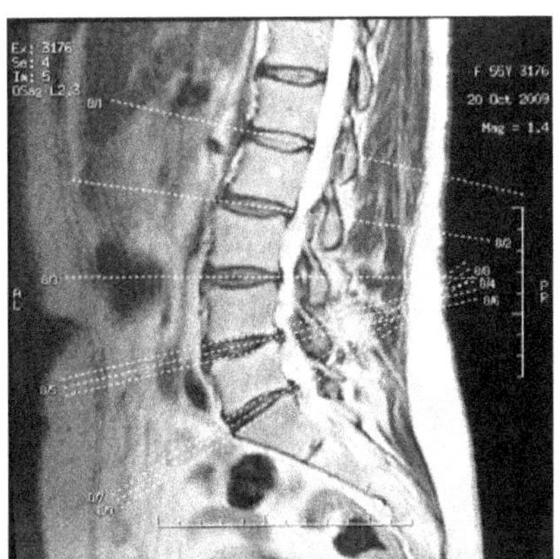

**Looking at an MRI of your spine will help
your surgeon determine if surgery is right for you.**

If you have had a history of cancer and there is a possibility that your cancer may have spread to your spine causing pinching of your sciatic nerve, and causing your sciatica, your doctor might order a bone scan.

If your bone scan comes back with a finding of a potential tumor in your spine, your doctor may order additional imaging to get more information on the spinal tumor.

Tumors of the spine may also show up on spinal x-rays and MRI.

Since sciatica involves pinching of a nerve, some doctors also recommend EMG and NCV testing. EMG stands for electromyography. NCV stands for nerve conduction velocity studies. EMGs and NCVs are usually done together.

They can help determine if there is a problem in the way your sciatic nerve conducts electrical impulses which can happen when a nerve is pinched. It can also determine if the muscles supplied by your sciatic nerve are working properly. This can help determine where the nerve is getting pinched or irritated.

The challenge with matching x-rays, MRIs, and other imaging of your spine to your sciatica symptoms is that research studies have shown that what you see on spinal imaging studies DO NOT always correlate with the symptoms of the patients.

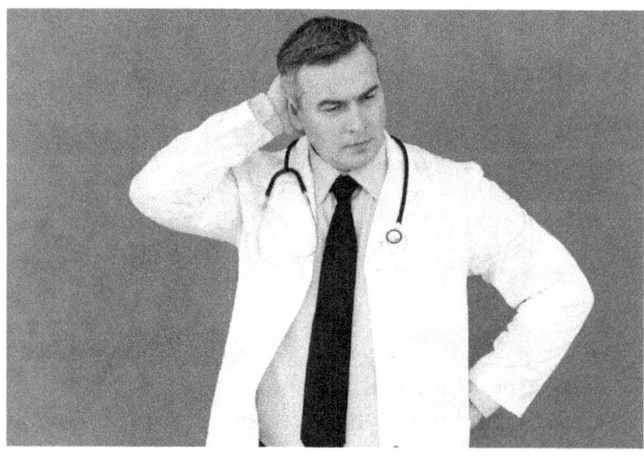

For example, researchers have seen people with severe spinal problems shown on x-rays or MRIs of their spine, and yet, these people walk around with NO symptoms of back pain, neck pain, or sciatica.

Researchers have also seen people with NO problems or MINIMAL problems shown on their spinal x-rays or MRIs that are experiencing severe pain and disability.

These studies have resulted in recommendations that doctors wait to order imaging of the spine – unless there is a good reason to do so. Some of the reasons to take spinal imaging right away include suspicion of fracture, tumor, infection, or cauda equina syndrome.

Other good reasons for imaging include having sciatica that is not getting better on its own or with conservative spinal care.

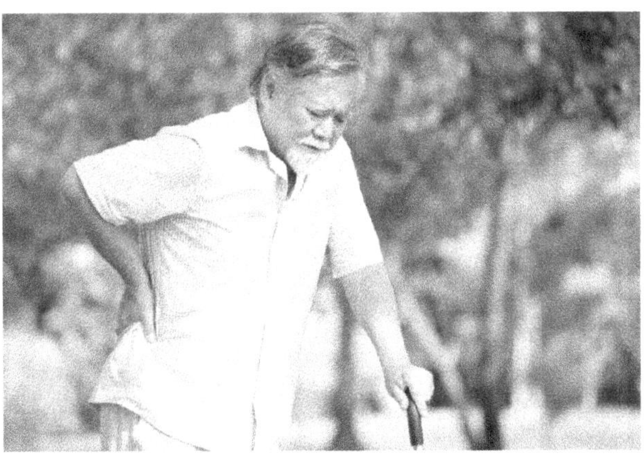

Also, if your sciatica gets progressively worse,
your doctor will be more likely to order spinal imaging.

Besides poor correlation of imaging to actual patient symptoms, many doctors wait to take spinal imaging because studies have shown that spinal problems often go away on their own within a few weeks.

If you do not want to wait for your sciatica to go away, and you insist that you want to see what is going on in your spine, your doctor will probably order spinal x-rays first. This is because x-rays are a lot cheaper for you and for your insurance company.

In general, x-rays can help your doctor rule out fractures, infections, and tumors. Although x-rays do not always pick up tumors that are small or hard to detect. X-rays can also show abnormalities in the anatomy of your spinal bones. Doctors can also use x-rays to diagnose spinal alignment problems.

For diagnosing spinal disc herniations, a spinal MRI is the imaging of choice. Again, MRI findings do not always match the symptoms of the patients, and MRIs are very time consuming and expensive. For these reasons, doctors must justify ordering spinal MRIs to the patient's insurance company.

Spinal imaging with dyes can show more detailed imaging of spinal disc herniations, but these imaging studies are more invasive.

Another tricky problem with spinal x-rays and MRIs not correlating to patient symptoms is that when you get spinal imaging done, this produces a record of your imaging results. This will become part of your permanent medical record, even if the spinal problems shown on the imaging are not creating problems for you.

In some people, having abnormalities and problems shown in the images of their spine becoming part of their medical record is not a problem. For some, it is problematic.

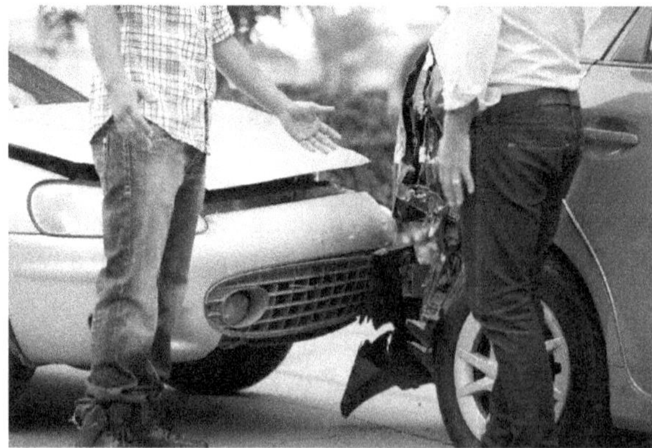

For example, if you get into a car accident.

In a car accident where it's not your fault, the insurance company of the person who hit you can use your previous x-rays and MRI findings as evidence that you had prior pre-existing medical problem in your spine.

The above scenario can lower the amount of settlement money that you can receive from the insurance company of the person who hit you. Hopefully, you won't get into a car accident.

Unless a patient with sciatica comes in with high probability of a fracture, infection, a tumor or cauda equina syndrome, many doctors who treat sciatica patients first treat their patients with conservative treatments to see if their sciatica will improve before they order spinal imaging.

If patients have a fracture, infection, a tumor, or cauda equina syndrome, most likely their sciatica will not improve with conservative treatment.

If a patient's sciatica gets progressively better after conservative treatment, there may not be a need for this patient to get spinal imaging studies such as x-rays or MRIs.

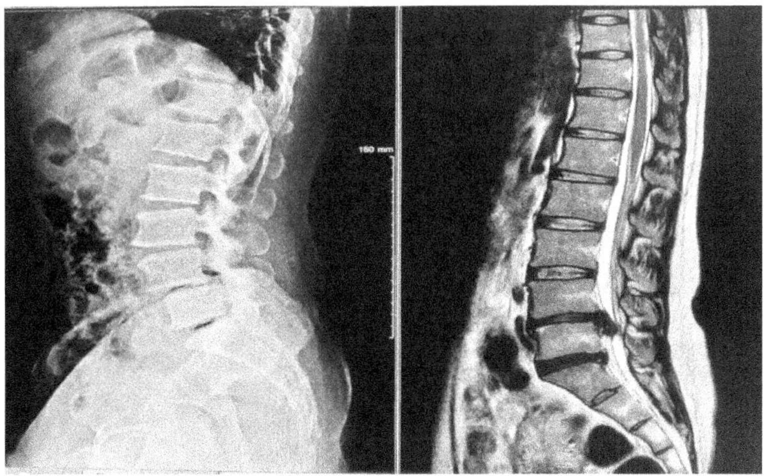

**When appropriate, do not be afraid
to get spinal x-rays or an MRI.**

Like other medical tests and procedures, doctors and patients must balance the benefits of getting spinal imaging with the drawbacks of having them.

Ask your doctor who is familiar with your health history and current medical condition to help you decide whether you should get spinal x-rays or an MRI.

5 THE #1 BACK POSITION
YOU MUST AVOID

What exactly can you do to get sciatica pain relief?

I am a chiropractor and I have a clinic in Soquel, California (USA) called the Back Pain and Sciatica Clinic. After over 20 years in practice, I have helped over 4,000 patients. Many of them suffered from sciatica.

The advice that you will get from this book is the same advice that I give to my patients who suffer from sciatica.

Before you follow any of the sciatica treatments that I cover in this book, be sure to consult with your medical doctor who is familiar with your medical history and your current condition.

First and foremost, let us stop the damage and stop your sciatica from getting worse. To do this, there are some things you should avoid doing.

The number one thing to AVOID is assuming the worst position for your back. Pay very close attention to this one.

Here is the #1 back position to avoid: BENDING over, while TWISTING your back, while REACHING for an object, while LIFTING or PULLING that object.

Take note of the activities that you do that require you to do this BAD combo move, and either avoid these activities or modify them.

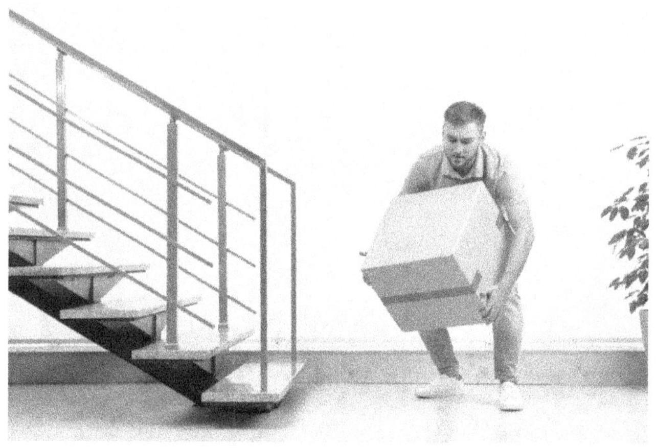

**This combo move is a KILLER
to your low back joints, muscles,
ligaments and discs.**

Many kids and adults do this move without knowing how bad this position is for their backs. When you are young and limber, you may be able to assume this back position without much pain afterwards.

As you get older, you will notice stiffness or pain in your low back while assuming the above position - or soon after.

If the object that you are reaching for and lifting or pulling is heavy, your back is in BIG TROUBLE. You may even hear a "pop" in your back when you injure your discs.

This popping sound is BAD NEWS.

Besides avoiding the bad combo move above, you should also avoid any back positions that make your sciatica worse.

When it comes to sciatica, "NO pain - NO gain", is NOT a good rule. Some people feel like the pain is creating a good stretch in their low back - not so. If you are putting your back in a position that makes your sciatica worse, you are probably doing more HARM than GOOD.

Avoiding positions that make your sciatica worse is a simple RULE OF THUMB that you should follow.

Following this rule of thumb will help relieve your sciatica and speed up your recovery. Ignoring this rule of thumb, will make your sciatica worse and will make your sciatica treatment NOT as effective.

The painful back positions to AVOID are different for different people. A sciatica doctor can tell A LOT about what may be wrong with your back by knowing what positions are painful for you.

What about moving your back
into different positions
to loosen up your back?

If done correctly, it is good to stretch and loosen up your back. But, do not move your back in the directions that cause pain – especially SHARP PAIN.

Knowing this information and following this advice can mean the difference between getting better and becoming a candidate for back surgery.

Avoiding painful back positions will not only help stop your spinal damage, but it can also prevent further injury to your spine. With this foundation, you are on your way to getting better.

Dr. John Falkenroth, D.C.

6 FIVE MORE COMMON ACTIVITIES YOU SHOULD AVOID

Be careful with coughing, sneezing, or bearing down when you have a herniated disc or a bulged disc causing your sciatica. Any of these three activities usually increases the pressure on your spinal nerve roots, which can make your sciatica symptoms worse.

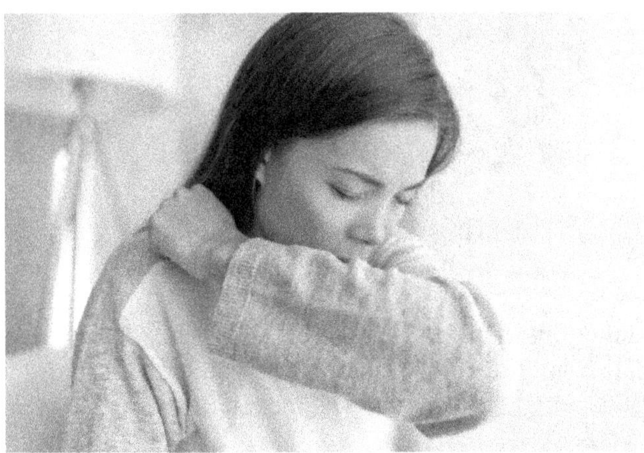

**Did you know that coughing
can make your sciatica worse?**

Another reason why your sciatica symptoms may get worse when you sneeze, cough or when you bear down, is because when you are doing any of these activities, you are usually leaning your shoulders and spine forward.

Just like coughing, sneezing, and bearing down, leaning forward causes extra compressive force on your herniated disc, which in turn causes extra compressive force on your sciatica nerve roots, making your sciatica symptoms worse.

You cannot always prevent coughing, sneezing, or bearing down. If possible, keep your back and neck in a neutral position when you feel the urge to cough, sneeze, or bear down.

This is easier said than done but try not to get sick when you have sciatica. Also, try not to get constipated.

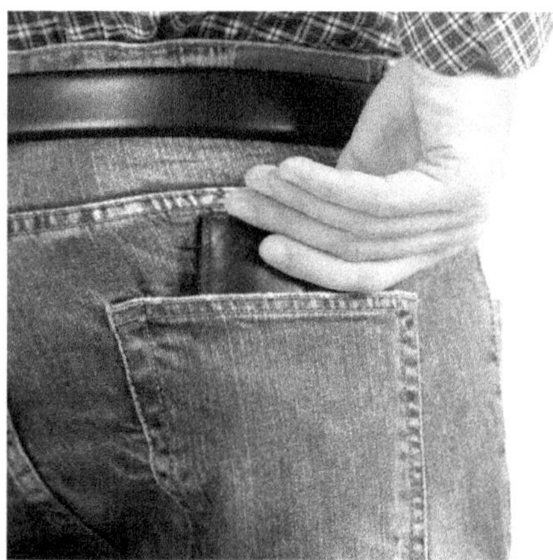

**Another thing to AVOID is
carrying your wallet or cell phone
in the back pocket of your pants.**

STOP doing this. This habit may be causing your sciatica - especially if your sciatica is on the same side where you carry your wallet or cell phone. If it is not causing your sciatica, it is probably making your condition worse.

Carrying your cell phone or wallet in the back pocket of your pants can irritate your piriformis muscle, which can irritate your sciatic nerve, since your sciatic nerve is located under your piriformis. It can also put direct pressure on the sciatic nerve.

You should also avoid sitting too long.

The habit of frequently sitting too long puts a lot of pressure on your low back discs and joints, dehydrating them, causing degenerative disc disease, which can lead to bulging discs or herniated discs.

Also, sitting too long can irritate your piriformis muscles and gluteal muscles. Irritated muscles in the buttocks can lead to an irritated sciatic nerve, which can lead to symptoms of sciatica.

As much as possible, minimize your sitting time. This might be easier said than done. Maybe your job or daily life requires you to sit for long periods of time.

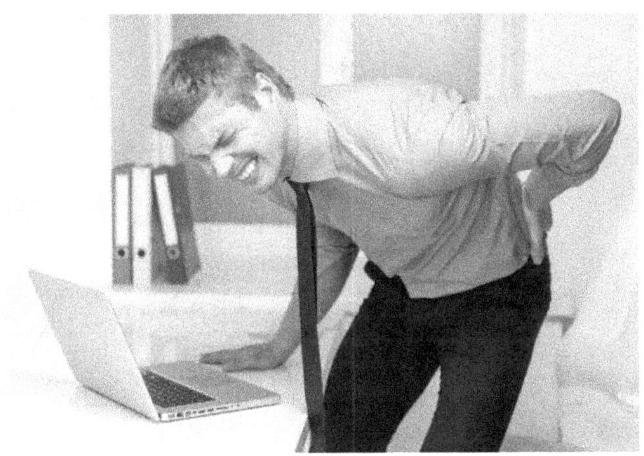

Prolonged sitting is BRUTAL to your spinal discs, especially to the lumbar discs in your low back.

If you absolutely must sit for long periods of time, there is a simple gadget that you can buy to take some LOAD OFF your low back discs while you sit.

This gadget will also help you maintain proper posture while you sit. What is this gadget? It is a backrest. Most people do not sit on chairs with adequate built-in lumbar support, so a good backrest is a MUST.

There are many backrests being sold today. Find the one that works best for you. Find one that helps you keep proper posture while sitting. Your lumbar discs will thank you.

When you find a backrest that works for you, sit with this back rest on your chair and see how much easier it is to keep proper posture while you sit. Make sure you sit all the way back in your chair so you are against the back rest and taking full advantage of the support.

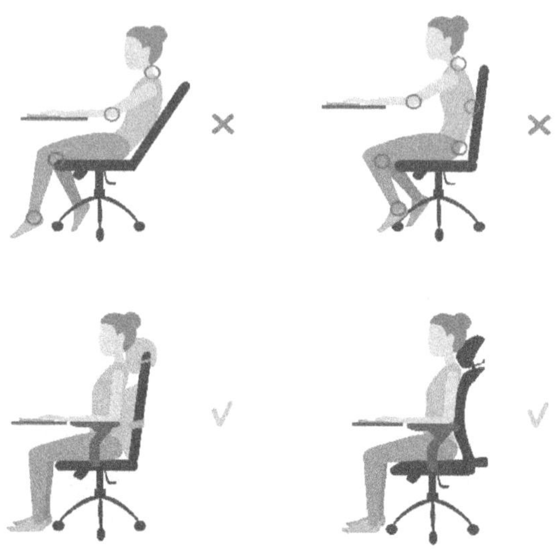

In my many years of helping patients with sciatica, I have tested many backrests on patients. I have narrowed down the backrest that I recommend to my patients to one backrest. This backrest works great for different sizes of people since it is adjustable.

My patients that buy this backrest often use it for their computer chair at home. Some patients buy a separate backrest for their chair at work. This backrest can also be effective in some car seats. If you get a chance to come by my clinic, you can try this backrest and see if it feels comfortable and supportive to you.

Keep in mind that using a good backrest does not mean that you can now sit for long periods of time. It just means that when you do sit, that your low back discs are not getting as compressed as when you sit without a good backrest.

Get up frequently and give your back a rest from sitting. It can be very useful to set a timer to keep you aware of how long you have been sitting and to remind you to get up and take a break.

Dr. John Falkenroth, D.C.

7 HOW SMOKING, ALCOHOL, AND EXCESS WEIGHT AFFECT SCIATICA

You probably already know that smoking is bad for you. When you suffer from sciatica, smoking is particularly bad in that it robs parts of your body of the oxygen that they need.

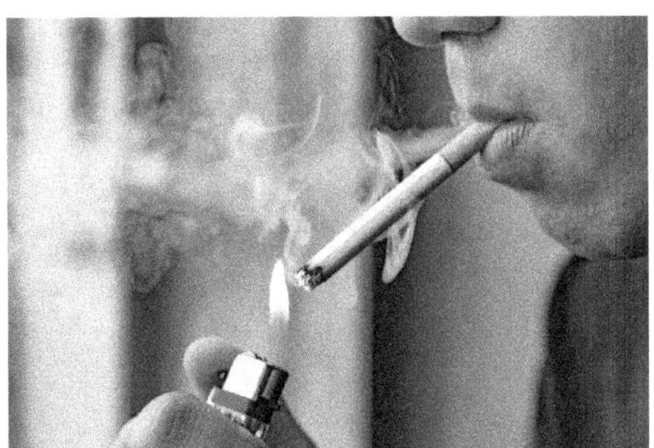

If you smoke, your lungs are not able to deliver as much oxygen to your body parts.

When you have an injury, like a herniated disc causing your sciatica, your injured body parts need as much oxygen as they can get to heal the damage.

Other healthy body parts may be able to deal better with less oxygen, but your injured body parts will have a harder time healing and may not be able to heal completely.

Drinking excess amounts of alcohol can also hinder your ability to heal from sciatica. Alcohol dehydrates your body. When you have sciatica, you probably have dehydrated, damaged, and bulging or herniated spinal discs irritating and pinching your sciatic nerve roots.

Your dehydrated discs need extra hydration and drinking too much alcohol will prevent your injured discs from getting the hydration that they so desperately need.

Also, drinking too much alcohol can damage your liver and make your liver not function as well. Your liver is responsible for filtering your blood and cleaning toxins out from your body. When you have an injured body part, your body will be producing chemicals to fix the problem. Some of these chemicals may end up in your blood and your liver needs to function well and remove these chemicals that can cause bodily harm.

If you are like many people who suffer from sciatica, you might be taking pain medications to deal with your condition – especially if your main sciatica symptom is pain versus numbness and tingling.

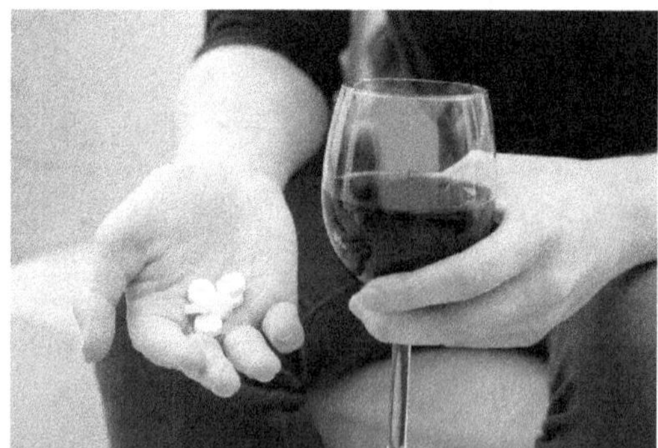

Alcohol can change the effects of medications.

That is why a lot of medications come with warnings not to take them with alcohol. If you are taking painkillers for your sciatica, either prescribed or over the counter, please do not drink alcohol with them – or close to when you take the medications. Alcohol also makes medications more toxic to the liver than they already are. Avoid drinking alcohol whenever you take medications.

Your liver is responsible for so many other functions in addition to filtering your blood. You cannot live without a liver, and a liver transplant is very complicated and may not even be available for you. Your liver cells do so much work to keep you alive and well. Do not kill them by drowning them in alcohol.

Now, let us talk about excess weight. I do not know if you're carrying extra weight, but you know if you are. If you are overweight, your spine must work extra hard to support the extra weight.

If your spine must support extra weight, your spine will break down faster and sooner than if your weight was within a healthy range. Your spinal joints are like your knee joints. Excess load makes them break down. Excess weight can lead to the formation of bone spurs, dehydrated and degenerated cartilage, and other problems. These are the same things seen in the spines of many people with sciatica.

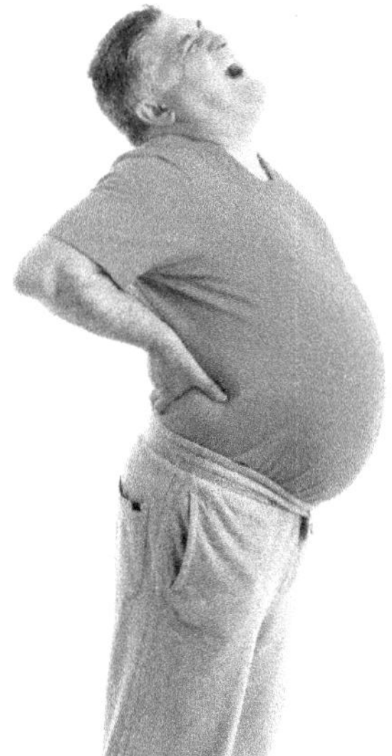

**Imagine the extra load on your
spinal discs if you are overweight.**

Most overweight people carry much more of the load in their abdomen, in front of their lumbar spine, compared to behind the spine. This uneven weight distribution causes abnormal pulling and excessive stress on the spine. This causes faster muscle fatigue and increased injury to the low back.

It is possible that your excess weight over time has caused your sciatica. Even if it did not cause your sciatica, your excess weight will make it harder for you to recover or heal from your sciatica. As much as possible, stay within the healthy weight range recommended for your height. It can help you recover from sciatica and can also help your overall health.

8 THE PROPER SITTING AND STANDING POSTURES TO RELIEVE SCIATICA

Now that I have told you what back positions to avoid, you are probably wondering what the best back positions are. Let us now discuss proper back posture.

According to Nobel Prize winner Dr. Hans Selye, M.D., *"The beginning of the disease process starts with postural distortions."* Let me show you how this statement makes sense.

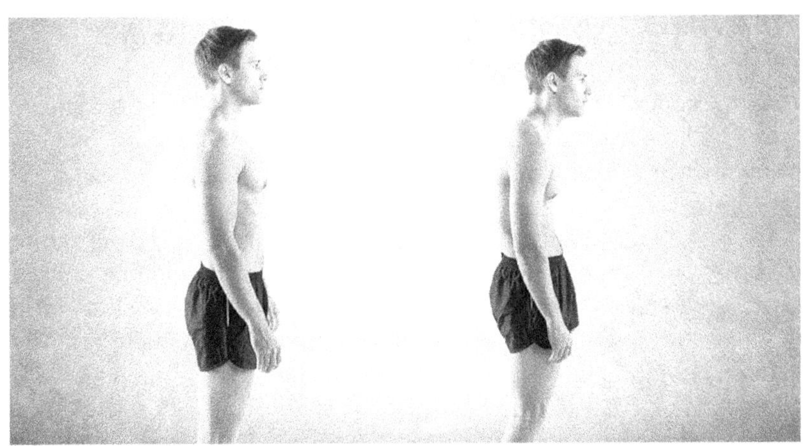

The picture on the left shows proper standing posture.
The picture on the right shows improper standing posture.

Find a mirror right now. Look at your posture in the mirror. Are your shoulders even? Are your hips even? How can you tell if your hips are even? Use your hands to feel your lowest ribs on each side of your body. Move your hands down until you feel the top of your pelvic bone. Look in the mirror and notice where your hands are.

Are your hands even in height or is one of your hands higher than the other hand?

Now have someone look at you from the side. Is your head sitting straight above your neck and in line with your shoulders?

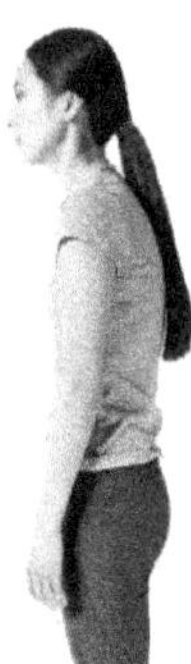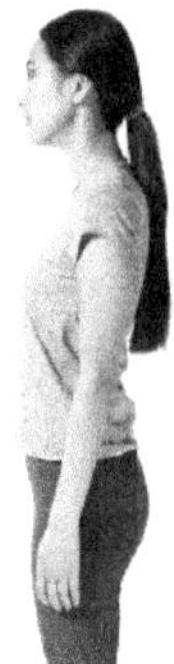

**Or do you hold your head forward in front of
your shoulders with bad forward head posture?**

With proper head and neck posture, the opening to your ear should be in line with your shoulders. Also, make sure you stand with your weight evenly distributed between both of your legs.

If you pay close attention, you may notice that you tend to put more of your weight on one leg when you stand. This chronic uneven weight distribution can create problems in your back joints, as well as in other joints in your body, such as your hips and knees, especially on the side that you put more pressure on when you stand.

When you must stand for a long time, and you feel the need to shift your body weight to one leg, be sure to alternate the leg that must bear more weight. It will also help if you stand on a cushioned surface, or if you can rest one of your feet on a small step or shelf.

Now let us talk about proper sitting posture. If you are like most people, you probably spend a lot of time sitting. Do you know what proper sitting posture looks like?

For proper sitting posture: put your head in a neutral position, where you are looking straight ahead. Make sure your head is in line with your neck, shoulders, and lower back. Also, BOTH of your feet should be comfortably resting on the floor or on a footrest.

DO NOT CROSS YOUR LEGS AND DO NOT CROSS YOUR ANKLES.

Crossing your legs or ankles will create stress on muscles, joints, and ligaments in your body. Your body functions much better in neutral, symmetrical position.

If you absolutely must cross your legs, do so at the ankles, but do not keep them crossed too long.

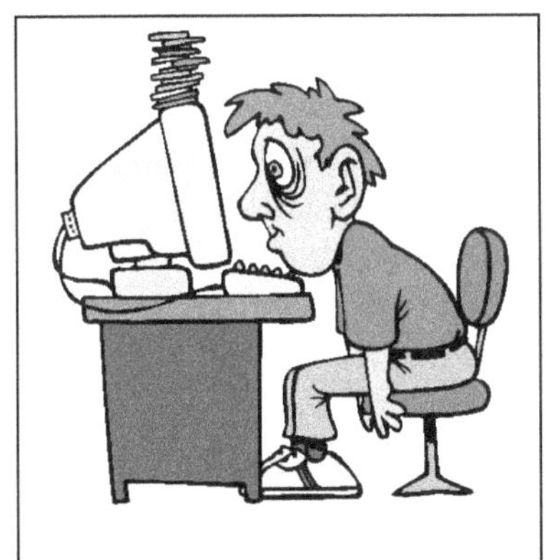

Bad sitting posture...

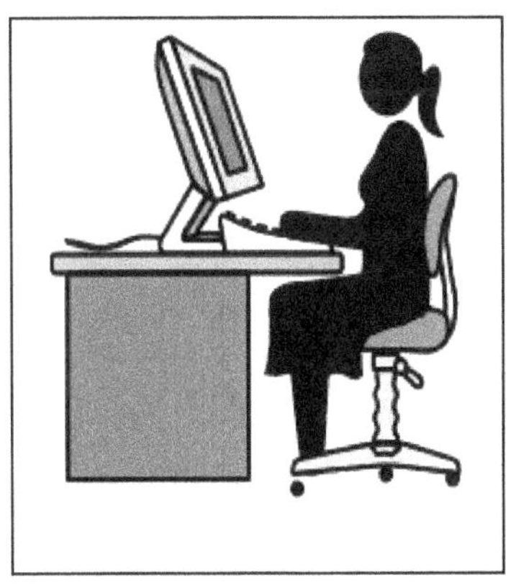

Good sitting posture...

Can you COMFORTABLY keep a good sitting or standing posture for 30 MINUTES? If not, you may have a problem in your neck or back that is preventing you from having good posture.

Problems like spinal misalignments, spinal arthritis, muscle weakness, and muscle spasms can make it difficult to maintain good posture. All these problems SHOULD be corrected right away.

Poor posture is associated with asymmetries in motion, leading to accelerated degenerative spinal joint pathology that will, in time, adversely affect the nervous system. (Koch et al, 2002)

This means that if you have poor posture, your joint motion will NOT be symmetrical. This results in faster wear and tear and degeneration of your spinal joints.

Since your spine has spinal nerves and a spinal cord that go through it, your spinal problem, caused by bad posture, will negatively affect your nervous system. Your nervous system is your body's communication system. It controls EVERYTHING in your body.

Therefore, good posture is not just good for your spine and your nervous system, but it is also good for the rest of your body, and for your overall health and well-being.

Let me show you how important good posture is to your overall health by demonstrating how posture affects your lung capacity.

1. Sit on a chair.
2. Take a deep breath.
3. Assume the best sitting posture position.
4. Take a deep breath.
5. Now slouch as much as you can or assume a bad posture.
6. Take a deep breath.

Could you tell the difference between your ability to take a deep breath and your lung's ability to get enough oxygen when you sit with GOOD posture versus when you sit with BAD posture?

Every part of your body relies on getting enough oxygen to stay healthy, to function well, and to NOT get DISEASE.

If you continue to sit with bad posture, this will reduce the flow of oxygen to the rest of your body parts that need oxygen. If not corrected, it is just a matter of time before your oxygen-deprived body parts will break down, and disease will set in.

Once again, as said by Dr. Hans Selye: *The beginning of the disease process starts with postural distortions.*

While this statement seems far-fetched at first, I hope you now realize that it makes sense. After all, Dr. Hans Selye, M.D. is a Nobel Prize winner. He MUST know what he is talking about.

Dr. John Falkenroth, D.C.

9 WALK FORWARDS AND
ALSO WALK BACKWARDS

Walking is one often overlooked activity that can relieve sciatica. This simple yet powerful activity is ESSENTIAL to your healing and recovery.

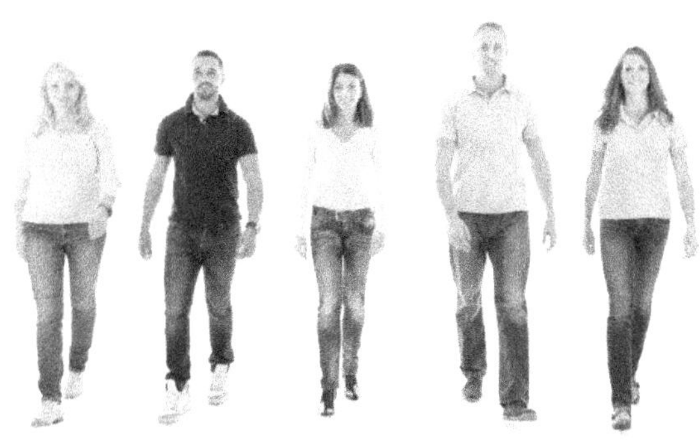

Walk a few steps right now with your arms lightly swinging by your side.

Did you feel your spinal muscles, ligaments and joints moving? You may not have felt your joints and ligaments moving, but you should have felt the muscles along each side of your spine moving.

Walk again, and don't forget the gentle arm swing. If you pay close attention while you walk, you will notice that your spinal muscles move in a synchronized way. Your muscles on one side of your spine will stretch while the muscles on the other side of your spine will contract.

This elegant contraction and relaxation of your spinal muscles is an absolute MUST for keeping your spinal muscles relaxed, flexible, strong, and healthy. Walking will also help prevent stiffness of your spinal muscles and keep them from getting spastic.

Walk again, with a gentle arm swing, and see if you can feel this synchronized contraction and relaxation of the muscles on each side of your spine.

Walking is also a good way to maintain a healthy circulation of blood and fluids in your spine.

Walking creates a POWERFUL PUMP in your spine that will help pump healing fluids and nutrients INTO your spinal joints, and pump harmful toxins and waste products OUT from your spinal joints - including your spinal discs.

Getting nutrients and hydration in your spinal joints and getting rid of toxins and waste from your spinal joints is VITAL to your healing.

Now try this - VERY CAREFULLY....

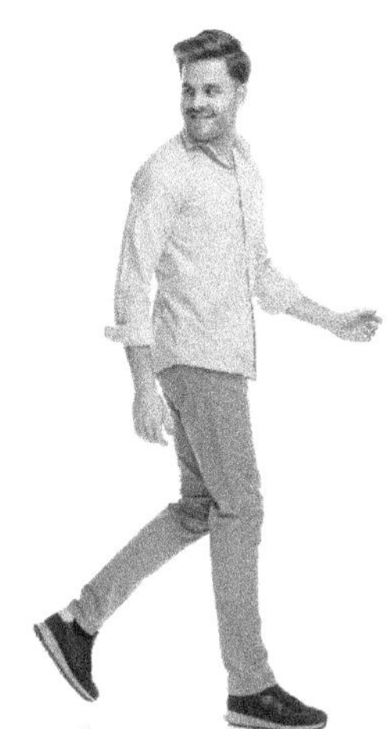

Walk backwards.

Be careful walking backwards if you have balance issues or if you feel weak or unable to do it.

Why walk backwards?

Studies have shown that muscles in FRONT of your lumbar spine are usually stronger than the muscles in the BACK of your lumbar spine. Since the muscles on the back of your spine are CRUCIAL for keeping your lumbar spine stable, they should be strong.

Walking backwards activates the weaker muscles in the back of your lumbar spine. This means that they will be getting more of a workout – making these muscles stronger. This will result in making your low back stronger and more stable.

Also, walking backwards stretches your hamstrings, which are often tight in people with sciatica or low back pain.

Walk backwards again. Can you feel your hamstrings getting stretched?

Sometimes, walking backwards alone can get rid of your sciatica, especially if your sciatica is from a simple muscle spasm or an overstretch injury. However, you must walk backwards for a few days to notice results.

So, whenever you are able, WALK forwards and backwards.

Do not overdo walking. Too much of anything, including something that is good for you, is NOT good. Walk forward first, then try walking backwards if you are able. Do plenty of walking with short periods of walking backwards mixed in.

If you are like most people with sciatica, you are probably NOT walking enough. Squeezing in more walking time during your day can help relieve your sciatica.

If you're not used to walking, or if your sciatica is severe, you may have to start walking on FLAT, SOFT surfaces such as grass or well groomed trails first, before you tackle walking on hills or on a harder surface like pavement.

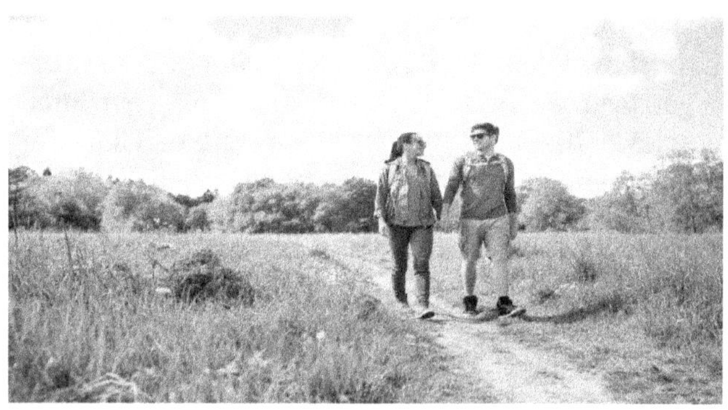

Be careful walking on uneven surface like the beach or unkept trails. Walking on these can make your sciatica symptoms worse, since your injured joints, muscles and ligaments may not be able to comfortably manage the challenging terrain. Also, you may not be able to handle the extra effort that these uneven walking surfaces demand.

If you are like most people with sciatica, you may be out of shape. You can START by walking around your house. If you feel the need to rest or to sit down after walking a short distance, you can easily sit down and rest.

If you are able, walk around your yard or outside close to your house so that you can get the benefits of walking and getting extra oxygen into your system.

Oxygen is VITAL to your healing and recovery, so make sure you get enough of it. If you are not able to be outside, open the windows in the rooms you are in.

If you are going to walk outside, away from your house, make sure there are rest stops along the way for you to sit on in case you need to rest. If you sit on the ground, it may be VERY difficult and very painful for you to get back up.

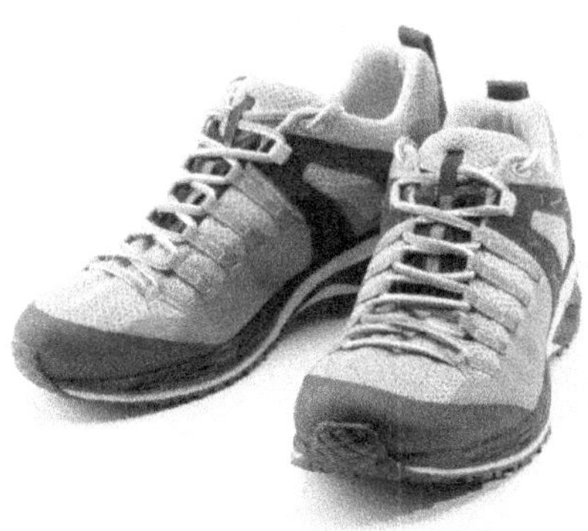

AVOID walking in heels or flip flops. Be sure to wear good, supportive walking shoes when walking. Not all shoes are created equal, so use walking shoes that feel comfortable to you.

If walking makes your sciatica unbearable, you should talk to your doctor about other things you can do to keep your lower back and legs moving.

If your doctor says that it is okay for you to do some walking, don't overdo it. Do not go beyond your pain tolerance. Do not go beyond your fitness tolerance either.

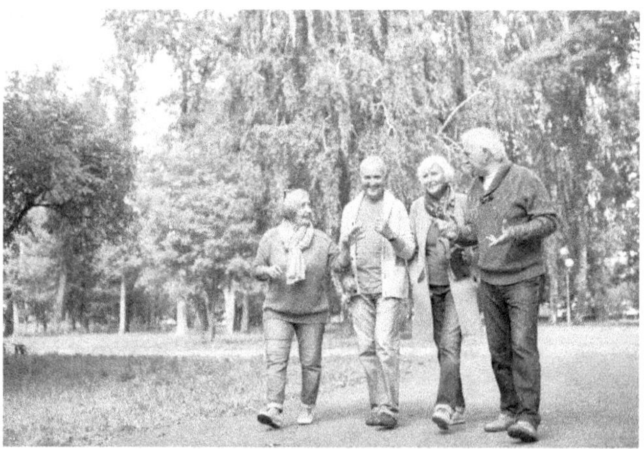

**If you have someone you can
walk with, walk with them.**

Walking with a partner is not only good for your back, but it will also be good for your emotional health. Take your spouse or partner or a healthy friend with you who can help you in case you need assistance.

Movement is very IMPORTANT for everyone, but especially important for people with sciatica - especially if they have had sciatica for some time.

Here is what typically happens to people with sciatica: Sciatica patients tend to develop a condition called kinesiophobia – a fancy word for fear of movement.

Unfortunately, if you restrict your daily physical activity, this can result in muscle weakness and loss of muscle mass. This can lead to a vicious cycle of more inactivity and more weakness.

Next thing you know, you will have poor tolerance of the normal activities of daily living, you might miss time from work, and you might also miss time with your friends and family. This can lead to depression.

Weak muscles can also increase your risk for flare-ups, causing more sciatica and other back problems. This situation can take you down a never-ending cycle of more dysfunction, stress, and depression.

Do not let this happen to you or to any of your friends and family.

10 DO YOU HAVE THIS FOOT PROBLEM MAKING YOUR SCIATICA WORSE?

Look at the bottom of your feet. Do you have good arches in both feet? Or do you have decreased arches or flat feet?

Now stand up. Is there enough space under each of your feet to fit 2 to 3 fingers?

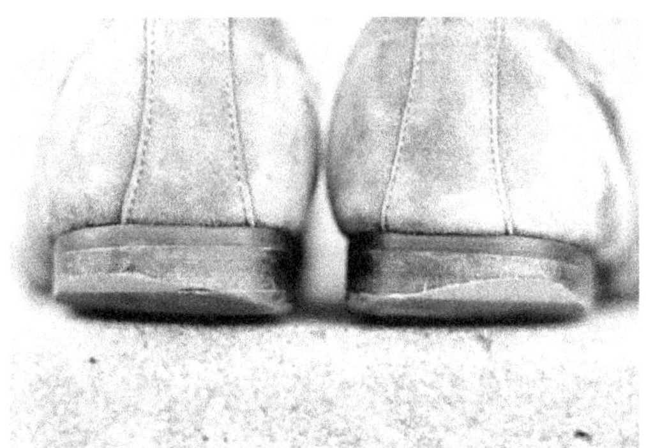

**Do you see uneven wear and tear on the
bottoms of the shoes that you normally wear?**

If you have flat feet, foot pain or uneven wear and tear of your shoes, problems in your feet may be causing your sciatica, or making your condition worse.

There are three arches in the feet. One on the middle of the foot, one on the outside of the foot, and one across the middle of the foot connecting the other 2 arches. The three arches in your feet should provide a strong balanced foundation for your feet, ankles, knees, hips, low back, and neck. These arches should also provide enough shock absorption to protect these joints.

Unfortunately, when the arches in your feet are weak, other joints in your body get forced to absorb the shock and the tension you create when you walk or run or when you stand.

This damages your feet, ankles, knees, hips, low back, and neck – and causes *early* arthritis in these joints.

Why do the arches in your feet collapse?

Here are a few reasons:

- Degeneration of the joints and arches in your feet as you age
- Past injuries to your feet, ankles, or knees
- Being overweight now or in the past
- Being born with foot alignment problems or having one leg shorter than the other
- Wearing shoes that do not fit well or don't have proper arch support now or in the past

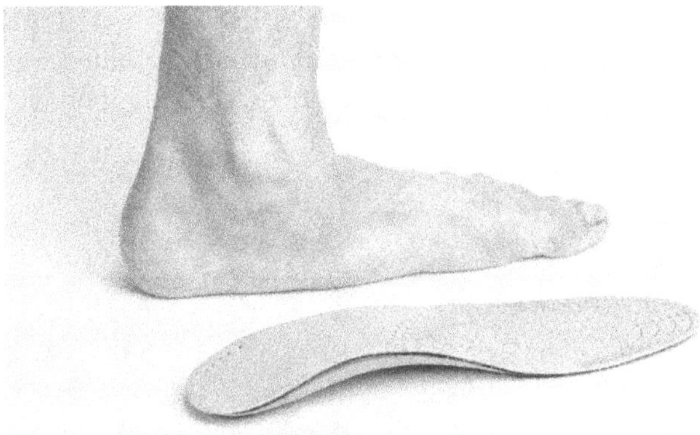

**If you have weak or collapsed arches in your feet,
consider wearing orthotics or arch supports.**

There are exercises that you can do to strengthen the arches in your feet, but most people do not have the patience or the perseverance to do these exercises.

Also, the arches in your feet are kept in proper place mainly by ligaments in your feet, and when your arches have collapsed, this can mean that your ligaments have been overstretched.

Overstretched ligaments are VERY difficult to repair. Even if you do foot exercises diligently, you may not completely repair your arches.

You can buy foot orthotics at stores. However, the problem with store-bought orthotics is that they're not custom-made for your feet. They may make your condition worse.

You can also get custom-made orthotics from a podiatrist.

A lot of my patients did not like the orthotics that they have gotten from their podiatrists, because some of the orthotics are made of hard plastic, which is very uncomfortable, so they end up not wearing them.

What I recommend to my patients with sciatica who have collapsed arches in their feet are custom-made orthotics that provide good support but are softer and more flexible than rigid plastic orthotics.

We perform digital foot scans on our patients to see if they have collapsed arches in their feet. The procedure takes less than 5 minutes, is easy and painless, and patients can see the results of their scan right away.

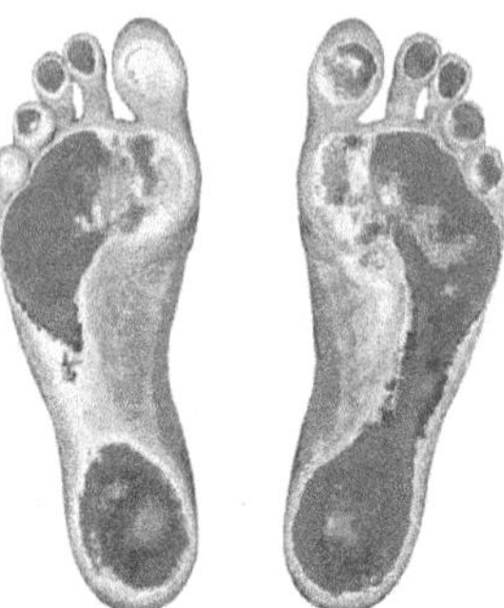

**A digital foot scan like this will pinpoint
weak or collapsed arches in your feet.**

If you choose to get orthotics, your foot scan gets electronically transmitted to an orthotics specialist. When we detect corns and bunions on a patient, we instruct the orthotics maker to design the patient's orthotics to make accommodations for the corns and bunions. This way, the orthotics maker can create a custom-made orthotics, made especially for your feet.

Orthotics come in different types of materials and finishes to fit your needs. You can choose the type of orthotics that you prefer based on the type of work or activities that you will be doing while wearing your orthotics.

Some people do not like wearing orthotics, because they are not used to having shoe inserts. However, after a break-in period, most get used to wearing orthotics and they like the benefits that they get from wearing them.

One of the main benefits of custom-made orthotics is that they help maintain your proper arches and help provide shock absorption when you walk or run. This protects your feet, ankles, knees, hips, back, and neck from further arthritic damage.

Patients who wear custom orthotics also notice dramatic improvements in their posture, especially when standing and walking. This improved posture also helps the health and function of their spine as well as reducing wear and tear on their spine. Patients often comment on how much taller they feel when they wear their orthotics due to the dramatic improvement in their posture.

Some of our patients have one leg physically shorter than their other leg. For these patients, we instruct the orthotics maker to build a custom heel lift based on our measurements.

Keep in mind that you can get a FUNCTIONAL short leg that is not anatomical and permanent. For example, if you have a muscle spasm on one side of your body, this can create a functional short leg.

In this case, the muscle spasm should be corrected, instead of adding a lift for the short leg, since the short leg is NOT a permanent anatomic problem.

From my experience with patients who have anatomically short legs, when they wear orthotics with lifts that correct for their shorter leg, they tend to keep their spines aligned longer between visits.

This also helps to increase the effectiveness of the chiropractic spinal adjustments and care that they get at my office.

If you have flat feet or collapsed arches in your feet, this may be making your sciatica worse. In this case, wearing custom-made orthotics may help you recover from sciatica.

11 USE THIS FORMULA TO DETERMINE
HOW MUCH WATER YOU NEED

In addition to walking and getting enough oxygen, drinking enough water is also very important for healing your spinal joints and discs.

You can walk all you want, but if you don't have the fluids to help nourish and hydrate your spinal joints and discs, and flush out toxins and waste products from your spinal joints and discs, you will be fighting an uphill battle. This will negatively affect your ability to heal and recover quickly and fully.

How much water is adequate?

Do you need 8 glasses of water a day no matter how tall you are or how much you weigh?

Here is a different suggestion as far as proper fluid intake that takes your body size and activity level into account.

Divide your weight in pounds in half and the number you get is the number in ounces (oz) of water and fluids that you should be drinking throughout the day.

For example, if you weigh 160 lbs., dividing 160 by 2 gives you 80. This means you should drink about 80 ounces of water a day.

If you are more active during the day, you will need more water that day. Also, if the weather is hot, you will need more water.

Making sure you get enough fluids will help you recover from sciatica. This is especially important for people with dehydrated spinal discs, which is often the case in people who suffer from sciatica.

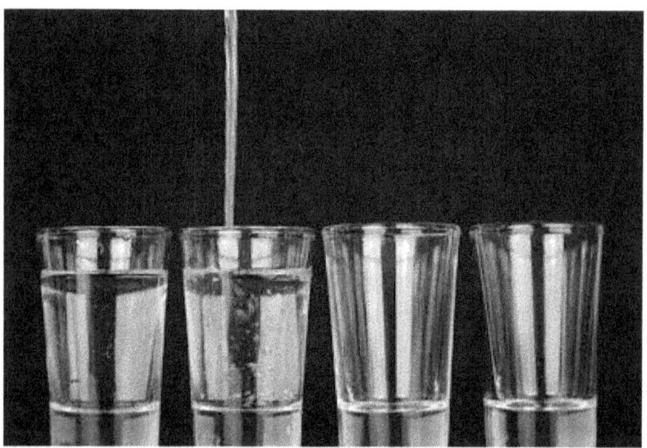

Water also helps flush toxic inflammatory byproducts out of your spinal joints and discs.

Make sure you are drinking good quality fluids and not the kind that dehydrate you such as coffee, alcohol, or soda.

You might notice that when you start drinking more water that you tend to use the bathroom more. This is normal for most people in the beginning when they increase their water intake. Soon, your body will adjust to your new hydration level and you won't have to go to the bathroom as often.

12 WHAT FOODS TO EAT AND WHAT SUPPLEMENTS TO TAKE

When you have sciatica, this means that you have inflammation in your body – in your discs, joints, nerves, muscles, and bones. Inflammation not only hurts, but also creates a cascade of events that can be very damaging to the inflamed areas.

As far as your diet is concerned, you need to not only eat healing foods that fight inflammation, you also need to decrease your intake of foods that increase inflammation.

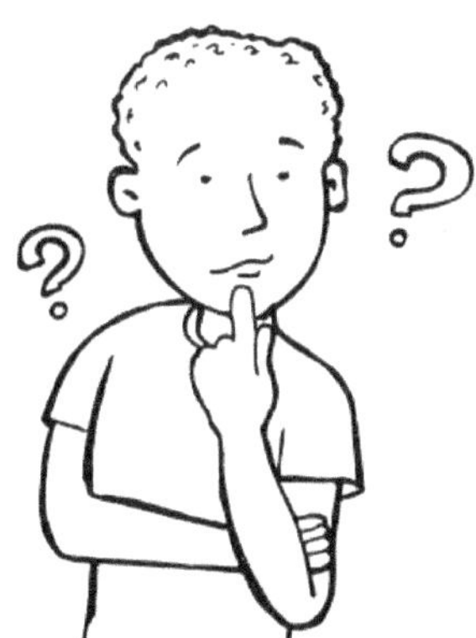

What exactly should you eat?

Different people have different body types and respond differently to different types of food. For example, certain foods may promote inflammation in some people, but not have inflammatory effects on other people.

To know exactly which foods negatively affect you, you will have to do your own research on how your body responds to different types of food.

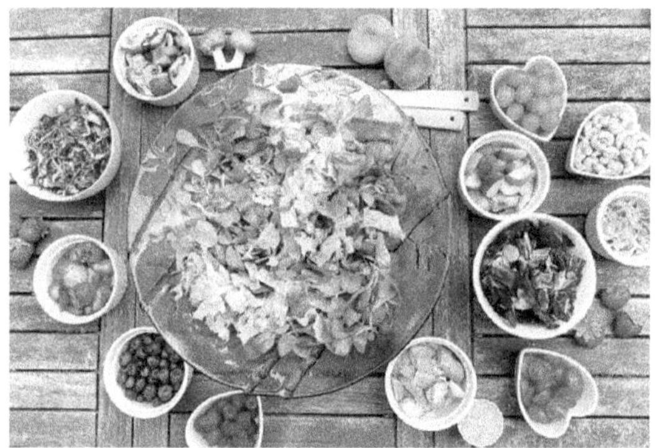

In general, plant-based foods such as vegetables, fruits, nuts, and seeds decrease inflammation.

On the other hand, consumption of animal products such as meat, cheese, and dairy products, tends to increase inflammation in most people.

Also, processed foods, especially ones with a high content of simple sugars, have inflammatory effects on most people.

It is very difficult for most people to make a complete shift in their diet.

The best method I have found, as far as patients shifting their unhealthy diets to a healthier one, is slowly adding healthier foods to their diet instead of forbidding them from having the unhealthy foods that they are used to eating.

Most people do not eat enough fruits and vegetables, so adding these to their diet can give them the anti-inflammatory benefits that people with a health challenge like sciatica desperately need.

If you are like a lot of people, you may not be a fan of fruits and vegetables.

You do not have to eat the fruits and vegetables that you hate. Choose the ones that you find yummy. There are many to choose from.

In general, fruits are easier than vegetables for people to incorporate in their diets. Most people find eating more vegetables harder to do.

If you do not associate vegetables with the word yummy, you may want to try using the seasonings that you find tasty, to make your vegetables taste good enough to eat.

Also, play around with how much you cook your vegetables. If you like your food crunchy, you may want to cook your vegetables only slightly instead of overcooking them until they are mushy and soggy.

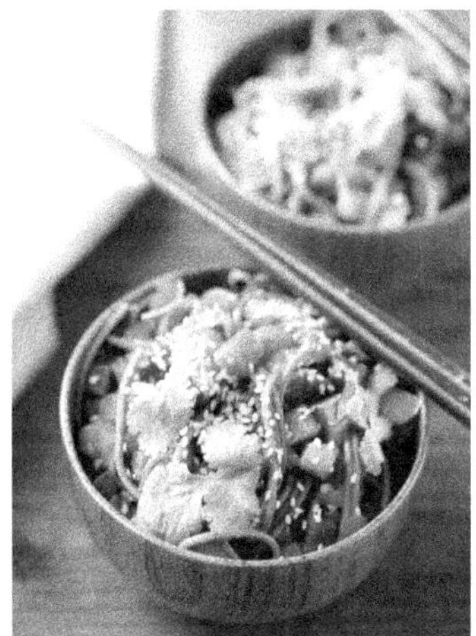

**Another thing you can do is to eat
vegetable dishes at restaurants.**

Since restaurants that serve dishes with vegetables have probably perfected their recipes, you may find their vegetable dishes delicious - changing your perception that vegetable dishes do not taste good.

Keep in mind that vegetables can also be eaten in the form of soups, sauces, and dips. For some people who are not used to eating vegetables, consuming veggies in the form of soups, sauces, or dips is an easier transition. Just be sure to consume a combination of cooked and raw forms of vegetables.

Look for sauces and dips in your grocery store with vegetables in the ingredients. Health food supermarkets usually carry them. You might be surprised at how delicious they can be.

You can also make your own. This can save you a lot of money. Get a recipe book or look up recipes on the internet for ideas. Also, if you find some from the grocery store that you like, look at the ingredients and see if you can recreate them on your own.

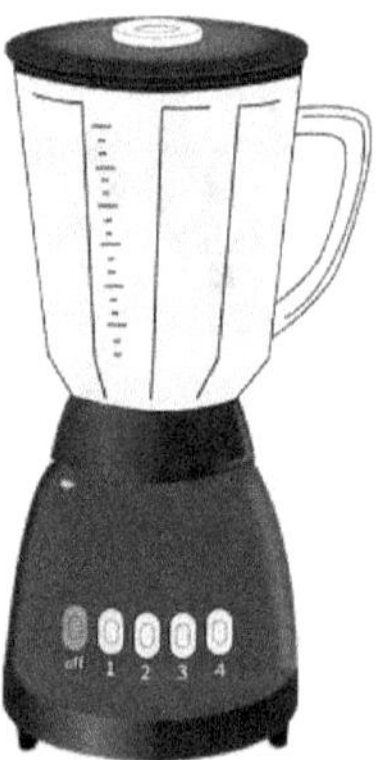

Making your own soups, sauces, and dips
will be easier if you have the right equipment.

Sometimes, you may only want to make a small batch, especially in the beginning when you are still experimenting. In this case, try a small blender or an immersion blender.

If you incorporate vegetable-based soups, sauces, and dips in your diet, you can eat a lot more vegetables than if you had to eat the vegetables in their whole form. Of course, it is best if you can do both.

Consuming vegetables and fruits in the form of juices can also help you get more of them in your diet. Just make sure you still eat the whole version of fruits and vegetables as well so you can get the beneficial fiber from them.

You do not have to give up on eating meat. You can still have your meat, but with added vegetables either on the side or incorporated in the dish, you will have a healthier and more balanced diet.

As I mentioned earlier, do your best to eat both raw and cooked vegetables. Cooking vegetables can change their nutrient content, so you may not get the same nutrients from the cooked version of the same vegetable compared to the raw or lightly cooked version.

Obviously, certain vegetables are not meant to be eaten raw, so it is okay if you only eat the cooked versions of these.

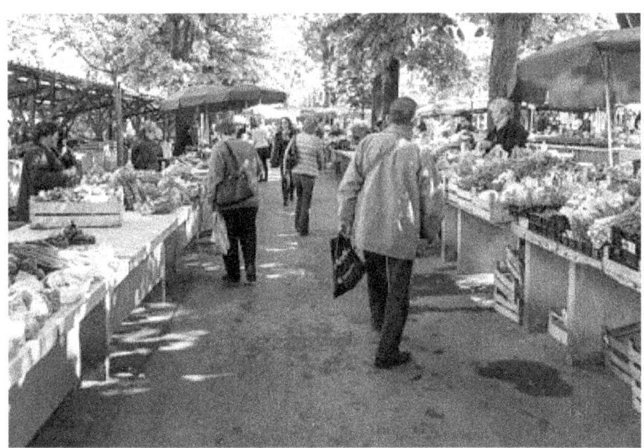

**Visit a Farmer's Market or a health food supermarket
and pick the fruits and vegetables that appeal to you.**

In general, you should eat the fruits and vegetables that are currently in season since these will be the freshest ones in the produce aisle.

Fruits and vegetables contain nutrients that are essential to keeping your body healthy and functioning at its best – vitamins, minerals, antioxidants, and anti-inflammatories.

Most people do not realize one other essential benefit of fruits and vegetables – their fiber.

If you are like most, you probably mainly associate the fiber in fruits and vegetables as beneficial for keeping your bowel movements regular.

Fiber also feeds the good bacteria in your gut. These bacteria are vital to your immune system and to your health. Your gut bacteria thrive when you have a lot of fiber in your diet, especially fresh fiber from raw fruits and vegetables.

Do not starve your good gut bacteria by not giving them the fruits and vegetables that they need to help them fight infections, diseases, and cancer.

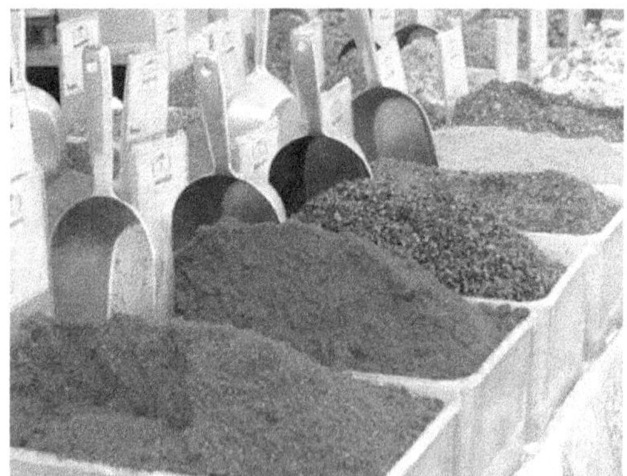

What about herbs, spices, and supplements?
What should you take for your sciatica?

Herbs and spices have been used for medicinal purposes for thousands of years - often with great results. Certain herbs and spices are used for healing specific conditions. I am not an expert on this method.

However, I can tell you that a lot of my patients with sciatica get great benefits when they take the turmeric and curcumin combo capsules that I carry at my clinic.

Not all supplements are created equal. Some have formulations or dosages that upset people's stomachs, so be careful.

Also, certain supplements, herbs, and spices can have harmful effects on some people, so talk to your doctor who's familiar with your current medical history before you take supplements - especially since a lot of these come in high dosages.

Keep in mind as well that certain medications and supplements interact negatively with other supplements, so talk to your doctor first.

If your doctor gives you the okay, maybe you can start by sprinkling small amounts of turmeric or curcumin in your cooking and see how your body responds to it.

In general, adding fruits and vegetables to your diet should have positive effects, but if you have certain conditions, or if you are taking certain medications, you should consult your doctor before making dietary changes.

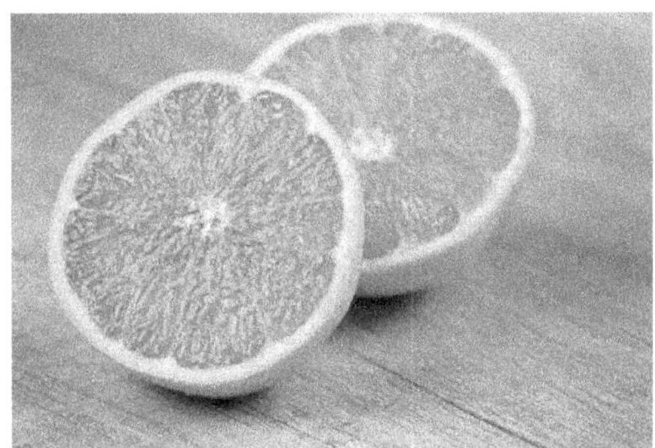

Be careful adding certain foods to your diet.

If you are taking medications for high blood pressure, you may want to avoid eating grapefruit, since grapefruit may negatively interact with your blood pressure medications.

To avoid negative side effects or interactions, always read the information that comes with the medications that you are taking and follow the instructions specific to each medication.

Also, you may have food allergies that you did not know about until you eat certain foods that cause an allergic reaction. Of course, stay away from foods that you know you are allergic or sensitive to.

Listen to your body. Introduce new foods into your diet slowly and keep track of how your body reacts to each new food that you incorporate.

Enjoy your fruits and vegetables and enjoy their health benefits

13 MAKING THE RIGHT CHOICE - USE ICE OR HEAT?

<u>WARNING:</u> Before you use ice, make sure you do not have a vascular or a neurologic condition that makes it unsafe for you to use ice. If you are unsure if you have this condition, ask your medical doctor.

If ice is safe for you, you should ice your low back to help relieve your sciatica. Ice is a great anti-inflammatory agent. This means that ice reduces inflammation and swelling.

Ice reduces congestion by PUSHING pain causing chemicals and fluids that build up when there's inflammation out of the injured area. Ice usually feels good, once the part that you are icing is numb. However, because ice is cold, it may not feel good in the beginning.

Heat does the opposite of ice.

Heat PULLS fluids INTO an area. Unlike ice, heat feels good initially. Unfortunately, people who use heat on their low back often realize later that heat made their back problem or sciatica WORSE.

This is because the additional fluid build-up in an already inflamed or injured area is kind of like throwing gasoline on a fire. It can increase the pain and inflammation and actually slow the healing process.

Where *exactly* should you put the ice?

Put the ice over the area of your low back that hurts. What if your back does not hurt? Is that even possible?

Yes.

Some people with sciatica do not have back pain. If this is the case with you, the problem is still most likely in your low back. You just do not know which part of your low back the problem is coming from, because your low back doesn't hurt.

Based on where your leg pain, foot pain, numbness, or tingling is located, a sciatica doctor can tell you which part of your low back your sciatica symptoms are most likely coming from.

In general, the problematic area will be in the part of your low back called L4, L5, S1, S2, and S3, since these are the nerve roots that form your sciatic nerve. These are located at the base of your spine where your low back becomes your sacrum and tailbone.

This is the area that you should ice.

If your sciatica is caused by a spastic, tight, or irritated piriformis muscle, ice the affected piriformis muscle in the buttocks on the same side as the sciatica pain.

If you have both low back problem and piriformis muscle problems causing your sciatica, ice BOTH your low back and your piriformis.

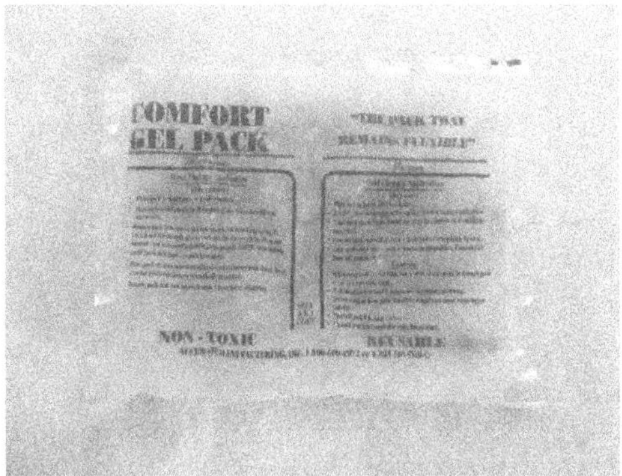

When using ice therapy, instead of using ice cubes, it is better to use moldable ice packs with gel-like material inside.

These moldable ice packs come in various sizes. Make sure you pick an ice pack that is big enough to cover your lower back and pelvic joints. DON'T PUT THE ICE PACK DIRECTLY ON YOUR SKIN.

Instead, put a thin piece of cloth, like your t-shirt or a thin towel, between your skin and the ice pack. You can have a thicker barrier if you are too chilled when using just a thin cloth.

DO NOT lie face down when icing your lower back. Lying face down is a very bad position for your lower back unless you have a special table, like a massage table, that is designed for laying face down. Instead, ice your low back while you are lying face up or while you are sitting.

How long you should keep the ice on really depends on your current condition and diagnosis. If you have a condition that is "uncomplicated," use the ice for 15 to 20 minutes every 3 to 4 hours.

In the beginning, when your condition is severe, you may need to use the ice pack more often. If you have recently inured your back or had a recent flare up of pain, then I recommend icing for 15 minutes every hour. Make sure you take the ice off after 15 to 20 minutes. If you keep it on for too long, then the body tries to heat the area back up which can increase inflammation. As your condition improves, you should be able to use the ice pack less often.

It can be helpful to apply ice to your lower back while doing other activities during your day. For example, you can ice while sitting down to eat, driving in the car, or watching TV. This helps to both make sure that you are icing often enough, and it also helps to take your mind off of any discomfort from the coldness of the ice.

Still, make sure that you are not icing for too long (more than 15 to 20 minutes at a time). Setting a timer is a good way to remember to take the ice off since the numbing of the ice can make it easy not realize how cold the area has gotten.

14 THE ONE RULE YOU MUST FOLLOW WHEN DOING SCIATICA EXERCISES

In general, if your sciatica is caused by a herniated disc or a bulged disc, DON'T do exercises that require you to bend your torso forward. Also, DON'T do exercises that require you to bend your legs upward.

If your sciatica is caused by referred pain from an irritated low back spinal facet joint or spinal arthritis, DON'T do exercises that require you to bend your torso backward.

Typically, when you do the exercises that are "BAD" for your specific condition, you will notice that your sciatica pain, numbness, and tingling will feel WORSE. Stop the exercises that cause this.

There is one rule you MUST follow when doing sciatica relief exercises: DO NOT do any exercises that make your sciatica symptoms get farther away from your spine.

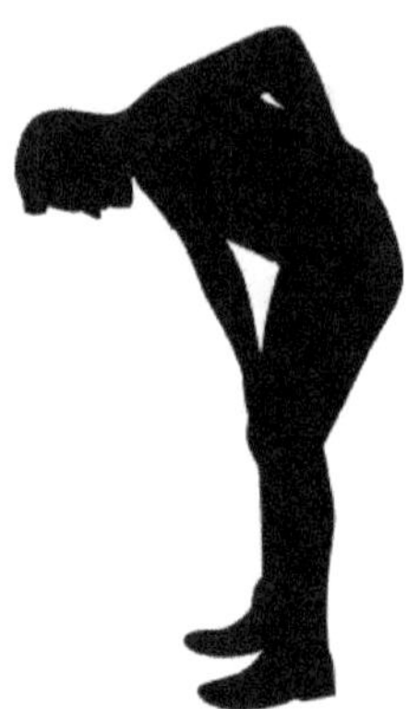

**With each sciàtica exercise you do,
pay attention to changes in the location
of your sciatica symptoms.**

For example, let us assume your sciatica symptom is tingling in your right leg. You perform a sciatica exercise. If during the exercise, you feel a tingling sensation in your right foot... or lower down in your right leg... STOP THE EXERCISE IMMEDIATELY.

Also, if you feel additional symptoms such as numbness, pain or burning sensation farther away from where your usual sciatica symptom is located, STOP the exercise.

If you also start to feel sciatica symptoms in your left leg, where you usually don't have symptoms, STOP the exercise immediately.

Even if you do not feel the increased symptoms during the exercise, if you feel any increase in symptoms AFTER you do the exercise, don't repeat the exercise.

When you feel sciatica symptoms lower down than where you usually feel them, or you start to feel new sciatica symptoms on the other side of your body, this means that you are making your sciatica worse.

Of course, if your sciatica symptoms do not move anywhere, but your symptoms get worse or more intense, then stop the exercise immediately.

Unfortunately, you may not always feel the worsening of your sciatica symptoms during exercise, but you may feel worse afterward. This is the reason why you want to consult with an expert who knows about your condition before doing sciatica exercises or sciatica stretches on your own.

Let us again assume that your sciatica symptom is tingling in your right leg. You perform a sciatica exercise. If during the exercise you feel a tingling or achy sensation in your low back and no more tingling sensation in your right leg, this is a good sign.

This can mean that the sciatica exercise that you just did may have decreased the pressure on your sciatic nerve or on the nerve roots that make up your sciatic nerve.

Keep doing the sciatica exercise that had this desired effect, but do not overdo it. Hopefully, you can find specific sciatica exercises that can move your sciatica symptoms closer to your spine, and eventually get rid of your sciatica symptoms.

Since I will only give you very basic sciatica exercises, you may not experience the desired effects mentioned above, but I hope you do.

Again, it is best to consult a sciatica expert who can help you determine the cause of your sciatica before you do any of these sciatica exercises.

Diagnosing exactly what is causing your sciatica is a VERY important step in putting together an exercise regimen that's specific to your condition and can help you and not harm you.

Another drawback of not having sciatica exercises specific to your condition is that it may take longer for you to get sciatica relief.

With that in mind, there are exercises that most people with sciatica can safely do. Again, if you feel SHARP PAIN in your low back, or anywhere, while doing any of these exercises, STOP immediately.

Also, if you feel your sciatica symptoms get more intense or move lower down your body from where you usually feel them, STOP immediately.

Not all sciatica patients have a low back MRI. If you have an MRI of your low back, you can ask your doctor to show you the exact location and direction that your disc has herniated.

Based on the location and direction of your herniated disc, your doctor should be able to tell you which positions might make your sciatica worse, and which positions should help relieve your sciatica.

It helps my sciatica patients a lot when I show them on their MRI which disc has herniated and in which direction.

Based on their MRI information, I advise them on specific back and leg movements that they should avoid, and movements that they should do to keep healthy movement in their spine.

15 THE 6 SCIATICA EXERCISES
I START MY SCIATICA PATIENTS ON

Stretching exercises work especially well when the cause of your sciatica is from a tight or spastic muscle.

Before we dive into sciatica exercises that may help you, be sure to follow the suggestions in the previous sections of this book. They will help make your sciatica exercises more effective.

PROCEED WITH CAUTION WITH THESE EXERCISES. If you do not know exactly which stretches and exercises to do, DO NOT do any. Guessing can hurt you and can make your sciatica worse.

Sciatica symptoms can be relieved by low back exercises. However, if you are getting debilitating SHARP PAIN with any of the exercises below, your sciatica may be beyond this point. You may have a serious condition that needs expert help.

Sciatica Exercise #1: Contract your abdomen

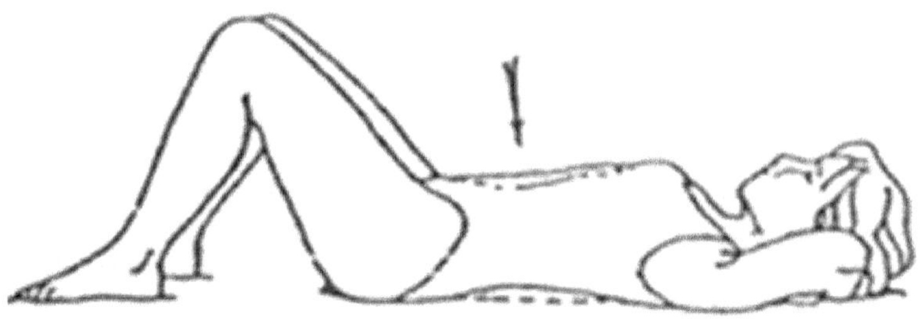

**Tighten your abdomen by moving your
belly button closer to your back.**

You can do this exercise while sitting, standing, or lying down. This means that you can do this exercise while you wait in line at stores or while you are waiting for someone.

You can also tighten your abdomen while lying in bed, sitting in your car, or sitting at your desk.

Doing this simple exercise often can help strengthen your abdominal muscles, which can help relieve your sciatica. This can be safer for you than crunches or sit-ups.

You do not have to hold your abdomen in a contracted state for a long time. Just do this exercise consistently. As a bonus, you may notice your waist size getting smaller over time.

Sciatica Exercise #2: Bend your knee toward your chest with your leg bent

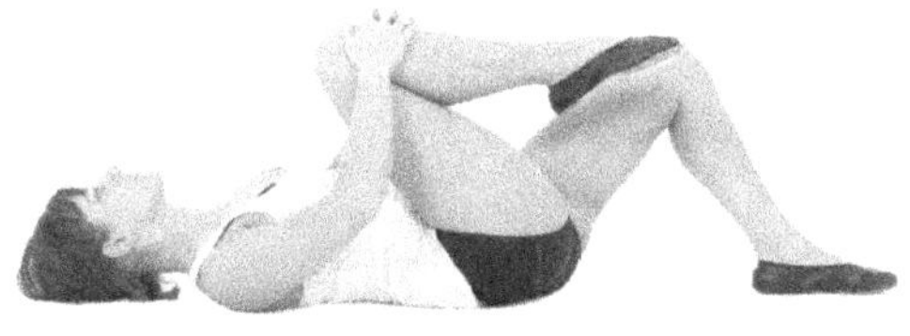

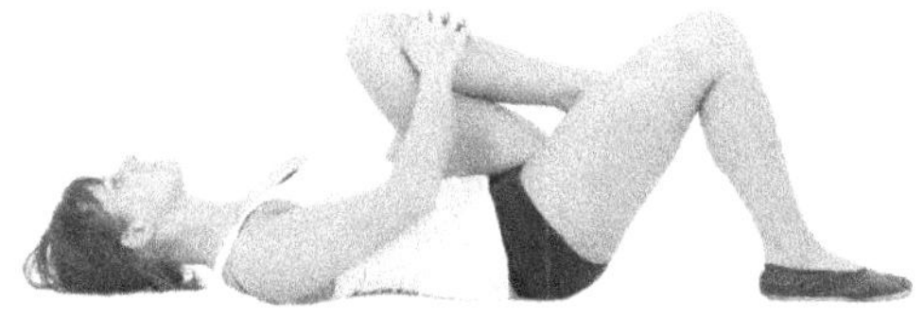

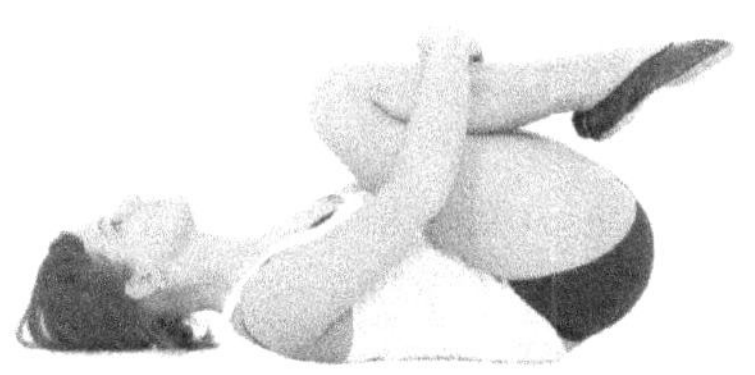

**Lie face up, bend one leg up to your chest,
then bring your leg back down.
Do the same thing with your other leg.
Then bend both legs at the same time, but only if you are able.**

You can use your hands to help keep your knees bent, but do not use your hands to help you stretch farther. You may "overstretch" and injure yourself. Do not overdo this stretch, and do not hold your leg in the bent position too long.

Sciatica Exercise #3: Stretch your Piriformis (Method 1)

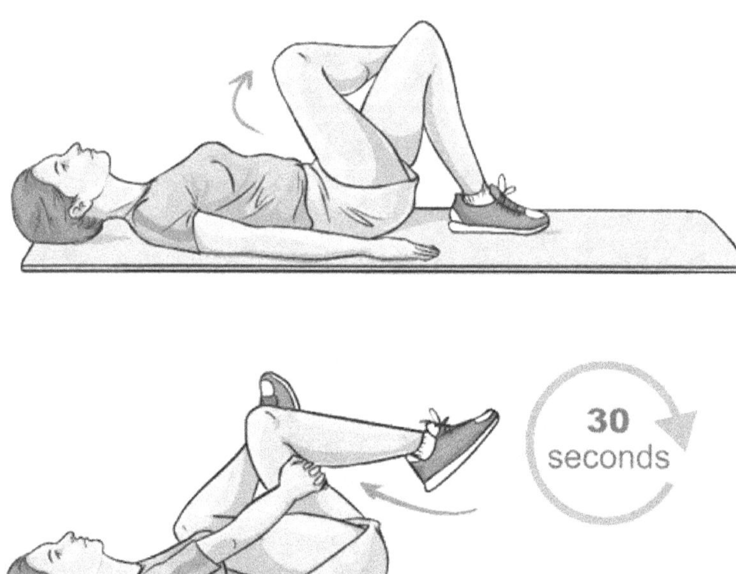

Put one leg over the opposite knee , then bend both legs
towards your chest. You can wrap your hands around
your top or bottom leg. Repeat with the other leg.

Sciatica Exercise #4: Stretch your Piriformis (Method 2)

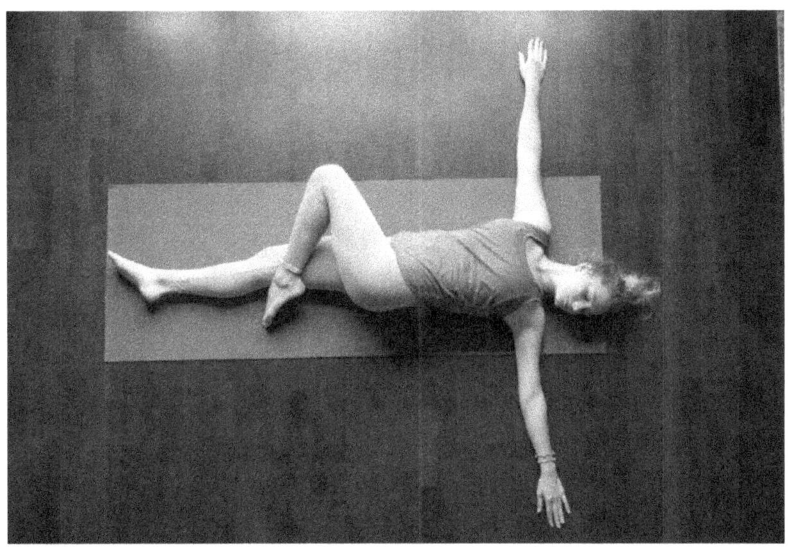

Lying face up, bend your knee toward your chest on the side of your
sciatica. Gently twist the bent leg to the opposite side which will
rotate the lower back. Do not overstretch. Lay your bent leg on the
floor. Be sure to keep BOTH of your shoulders touching the ground.

You can choose the piriformis stretching exercise that works best for
you, or you can do both methods. If you have very tight or spastic
piriformis, you should feel your piriformis get stretched when you do the
two exercises above.

If you have a tight hip, you will feel it when you do sciatica exercise
#4. If your hips are tight, you also need to loosen up your hip, since it
may be complicating your sciatica. I usually give my patients specific
exercises for a tight hip

Sciatica Exercise #5: Hip Flexor Stretch/ Gentle Lunge

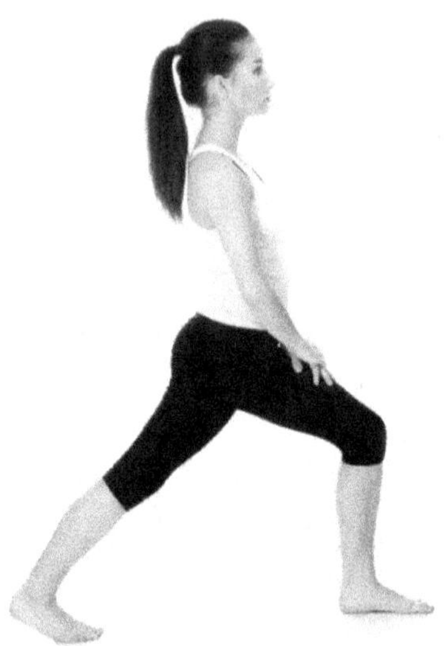

**While standing, take a small step forward (about 12 inches).
While keeping your back upright and straight and your tailbone
tucked in, move your torso gently forward until you feel a gentle
stretch in the front of the hip of the back leg.
Repeat on the opposite side with the other leg in front.**

Sciatica Exercise #6: Move and stretch your lower back

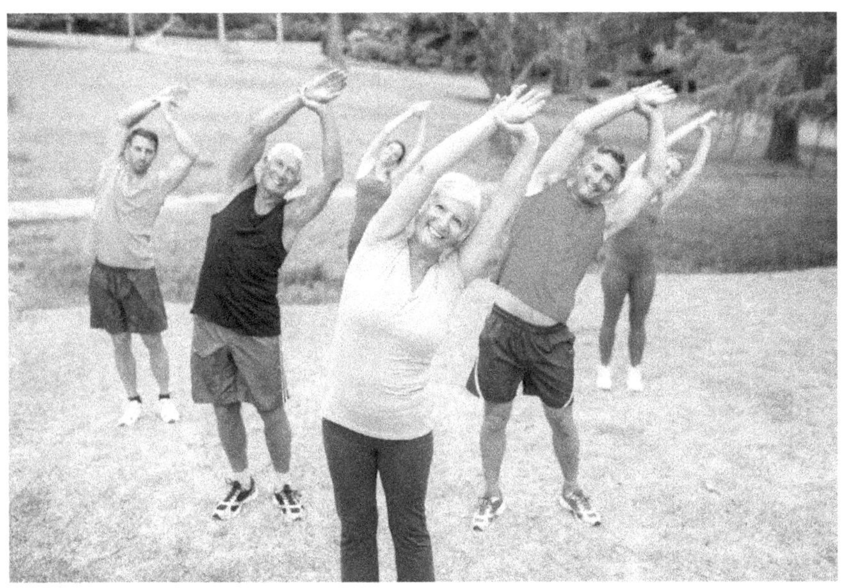

While keeping your back straight, bend your back forward. Then backward. Then lean right. Then lean left. Then move your upper body to look over your RIGHT shoulder. Then move your upper body to look over your LEFT shoulder.

Do these stretches CAREFULLY. Do not move your back quickly. Move it nice and slow. You can stretch your back while sitting or while standing.

If your sciatica is caused by a herniated or bulged low back disc, you may find bending forward painful. If so, DON'T bend forward.

You may also find bending to one side painful. If so, DON'T bend to the side that's painful.

If your herniated disc or bulged disc is severe, you may not find a comfortable position. All positions and all movements may hurt.

If your sciatica is caused by a referred pain from an inflamed facet joint in your low back, you may find bending backward painful. If so, DON'T bend backward.

Keep in mind that even if your pain or symptoms get worse when you bend backward, it is still possible that your sciatica is caused by a herniated disc.

This can mean that in addition to your herniated low back disc, that you may also have facet syndrome or facet arthritis complicating your sciatica. This is common in the elderly.

To understand why this is the case, be sure to read the section in this book titled, *"How Aging Wreaks Havoc on Your Spine."*

With the exercises and stretches that I discussed in this section, you are probably asking the following questions:

- How long should I hold each position?
- How many repetitions should I do?
- How many times a day should I do them?
- When should I do these exercises?

How long should you hold each position?

Start holding each position for 2-3 seconds. As you get stronger, you may be able to hold them longer, but don't overdo it.

How many repetitions should you do?

Do as many as you can comfortably handle. Again, be careful not to overdo it. Start with 3-5 reps - less if you are not able to. Do more repetitions as you are able.

In sciatica exercise #1, contracting your abdomen, you should be able to do a lot of reps of this exercise compared to the other sciatica exercises I covered.

When is the best time to do these sciatica exercises?

Do them at a time that works best for you. Also, when you start to feel your sciatica symptoms getting worse, stop what you are doing and do these sciatica exercises. This can help your keep your sciatica from getting *much* worse.

I understand that sometimes your back may start hurting at work where the floor is not clean enough to lie down on.

You can bring a yoga mat or large towel to work or leave one in your car in case you need it. The mat you use doesn't have to be fancy – you just need a clean surface.

Also, get a mat or towel with some cushion, especially if the floor at your work is hard like cement or hardwood. A cushioned mat will help make the exercises more comfortable.

DON'T do these exercises first thing in the morning. Your muscles and ligaments will not be warmed up, and you will be more prone to injury.

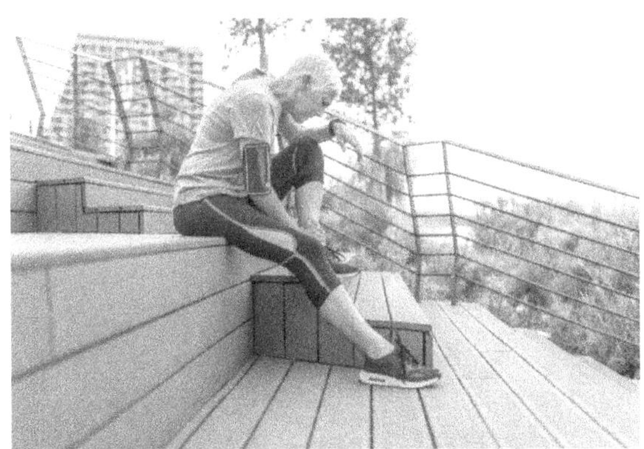

**Do not do these sciatica exercises
when you are EXHAUSTED.**

When you are extremely tired, your muscles and ligaments will have less strength to protect your joints if you overstretch.

How many times a day should you do these sciatica exercises?

Twice a day works well for most people. It is better to do these exercises more often throughout the day, instead of overdoing them with excessive repetitions or by holding the positions too long.

After you do the sciatica exercises, you might feel sore in certain areas. Ice these sore areas and be sure to follow the icing instructions that I covered in the previous section.

16 HOW TO KEEP YOUR SPINE ALIGNED AND MOVING PROPERLY

In an earlier chapter, we talked about how misaligned spinal joints that do not move properly can cause sciatica or make sciatica worse.

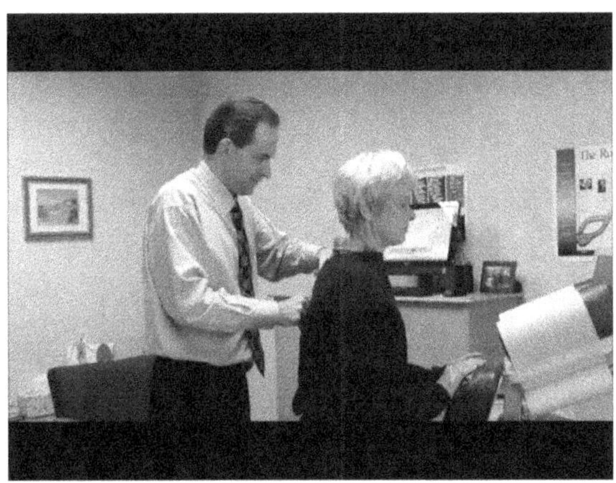

**One of the most important things you can do
to relieve your sciatica is to make sure to keep
your spine aligned and moving properly.**

You can do the spinal stretches and exercises that I mentioned earlier to help keep your spine aligned and moving. However, there are times when one or more joints in your spine can get misaligned, stiff, or stuck in place.

Carefully move your back in different directions right now - forwards, backwards, bending left, bending right, looking over your left shoulder, then looking over your right shoulder.

Did you notice certain areas or spots in your back that felt tight, sore, or painful when you tried these movements? These areas of your spine may have misaligned bones or joints that do not move properly.

If you are able, use the tips of your fingers to feel the muscles on each side of your spine where you noticed tightness, soreness, or pain when you moved your back in different directions.

Feel the muscles on each side closest to your spine.

When you felt your back muscles, did you notice spots that felt tender? Did you notice tight muscles? These areas may have misaligned or stuck spinal joints, spinal arthritis, herniated discs, bulged discs, or other problems.

Just like other parts of your body need regular check-ups and tune-ups, your spine also needs to be checked and re-aligned on a regular basis.

We use our spine every day and things such as lifting, pulling, bending, prolonged sitting, bad posture, and lack of movement can make our spinal joints misaligned or stuck.

When it comes to detecting and correcting spinal joints that are misaligned or stuck, my colleagues and I... chiropractors... do this best.

Chiropractors use various treatment methods to treat patients.

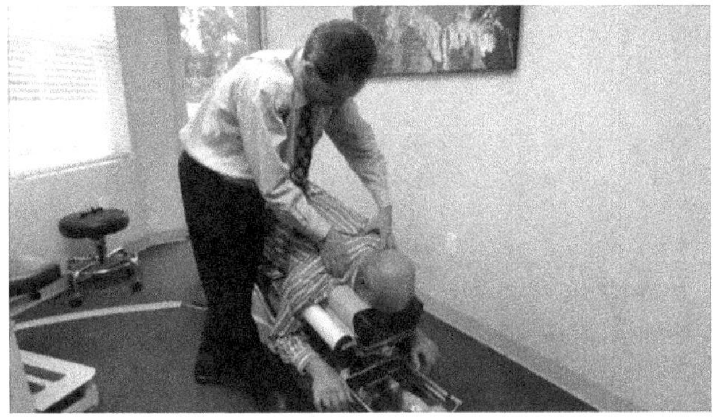

Some chiropractors use traditional hands-on treatments.

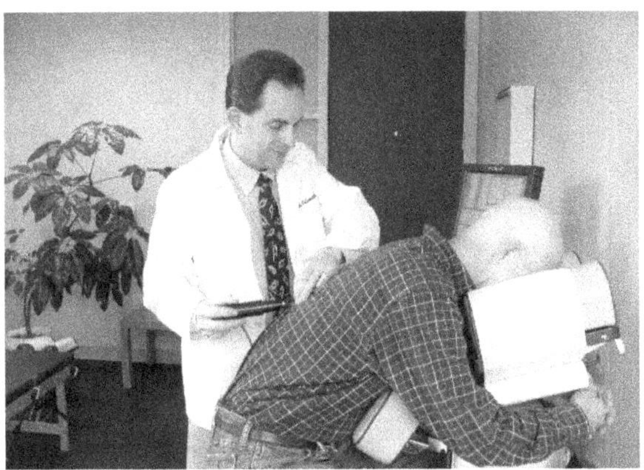

**Some chiropractors use instrument-guided
treatments that do not require cracking,
popping, or twisting of your spine.**

Since chiropractors use different treatment methods, this can create confusion as to who to go to when sciatica patients are looking for a chiropractor.

Because chiropractors have different ways that they treat patients, chiropractic patients can choose the treatment method that works best for them.

If one chiropractic method does not work for you, try another one.

Keep trying different chiropractic treatment methods until you find a method or a chiropractor that helps you with your sciatica.

Do not give up because you went to one chiropractor and you did not like their treatment method, office environment, or personality. If you went to a dentist and you did not like them, would you stop going to the dentist for the rest of your life? What would happen to your teeth if you did this?

Keeping your spinal joints aligned properly and moving normally, will not only help relieve your sciatica, but can also help prevent future spinal problems from showing up later. How?

Each joint in your spine is indirectly connected to other joints in the spine… especially the ones directly above and directly below each spinal joint. When you have spinal misalignment or abnormal spinal motion, the joints above and below the problem joint will need to compensate to keep the alignment and motion of your spine as close to normal as possible.

These joints will start to have problems if they must keep compensating for the problematic joint. Then, the bones and joints around them will also need to compensate causing new problems in these areas as well.

If not stopped, you will have a vicious cycle of spinal joint degeneration happening up and down your spine.

You may notice that over time, your joints above and below the initial problem area will also develop degenerative joint problems.

This is one of the reasons why people with sciatica or low back problems often also end up experiencing midback problems and neck problems.

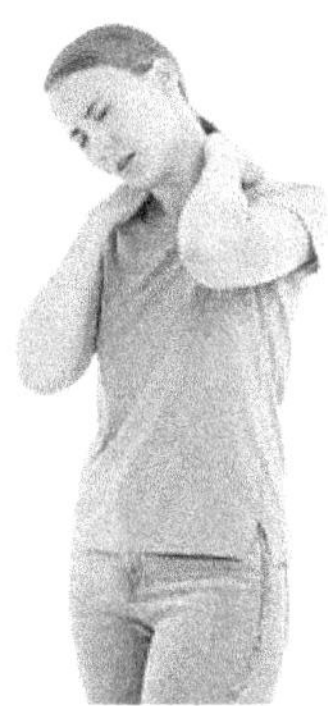

**It is common for people with sciatica
to also develop neck pain as a side effect.**

At my chiropractic clinic, I use both traditional hands on treatment methods and computer-guided instrument methods.

Some of my patients, especially the older ones, do not like or cannot tolerate manual chiropractic treatments. These patients love the computer -guided instrument methods.

My younger patients, especially those used to the more powerful adjustment methods, love the traditional hands-on chiropractic treatments.

Keep in mind that the hands-on treatments do not have to be forceful. An experienced practitioner can modify their hands-on treatments to deliver gentle treatments to patients who prefer or require a gentler approach.

Also keep in mind that chiropractors prefer to treat different types of conditions and different types of patients. For example, there are chiropractors who prefer to treat children or athletes and others that work with more seniors.

When you look for a chiropractor to help you with your sciatica, be sure to ask them if they treat sciatica patients. Also, ask about their years of experience in treating patients with sciatica.

17 CAN MASSAGE HELP SCIATICA?

Just like it is important to get treated by a chiropractor who treats lots of sciatica patients, it is also important to get massaged by a massage therapist who has experience in treating sciatica patients.

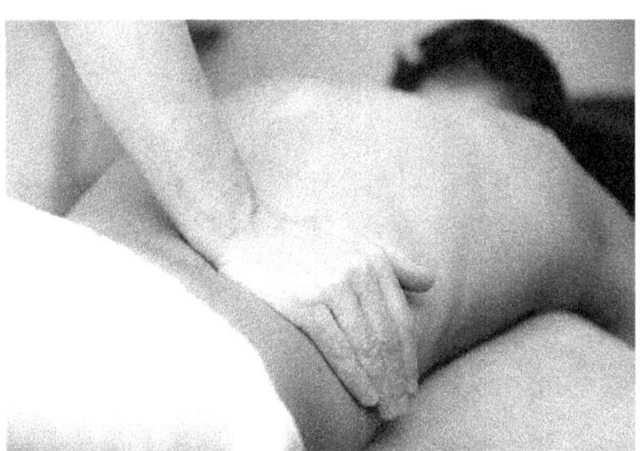

**Massage can help relax your tight muscles
that may be causing or contributing to your sciatica.**

Since one of the causes of sciatica is a tense piriformis muscle, then relaxing this tense muscle can relieve your sciatica.

However, if your piriformis muscle is in acute spasm, not just tight or tense, you may find that that massage is very painful.

Have you ever had a charley horse or muscle cramp? If you did, would you have liked having someone dig hard into your cramping calf muscle and try to relax your spastic muscle?

Probably not. You would have screamed in pain or kicked them with your other foot if they did this.

A much better approach is to have them help you by slowly flexing your foot up on the side of the charley horse... or by massaging your foot... or by massaging around your knees... or by VERY gently massaging your calf. If you are able, you can also do these yourself.

An experienced massage therapist should know not to directly dig in and do a deep tissue massage on the muscle belly of an injured muscle with an active acute muscle spasm.

Once your piriformis is not in acute spasm, your massage therapist should be able to massage and relax the muscle, thus relieving pressure on your sciatic nerve.

Massage can also relieve tight muscles in your back. Most sciatica patients have tight or spastic lower back muscles.

Massage not only helps relax your tight muscles, but massage can also release "feel good" chemicals called endorphins. These endorphins can help relieve your sciatica, especially if your main sciatica symptom is pain.

Again, the key is to find a massage therapist experienced in treating patients with sciatica. Otherwise, massage may harm you and make your sciatica symptoms worse.

If massage COMPLETELY relieves your sciatica symptoms, then your tight piriformis may have been the cause of your sciatica. You belong in the more fortunate group of sciatica sufferers.

Most sciatica is caused by a herniated disc or a bulging disc in the low back pinching or irritating the sciatic nerve Massage alone cannot fix this. You need to get the pressure off your pinched nerve as soon as possible.

18 PAINKILLERS, MUSCLE RELAXANTS, AND ANTI-INFLAMMATORY DRUGS

If you go to the emergency room or to your doctor complaining of sciatica, and they don't find fractures, tumors, infections, or other serious problems that need immediate attention, you will usually come home with a prescription for painkillers, anti-inflammatories, or muscle relaxants.

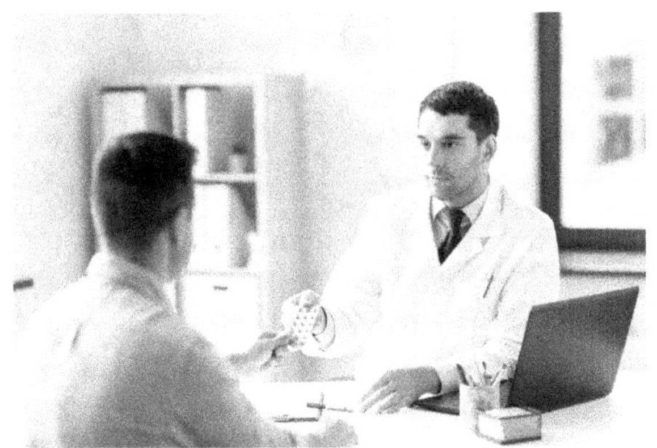

Of course, the medication they prescribe you will depend on your condition.

Some doctors may also write you a prescription for antidepressants. Why? First, because people with sciatica can get depressed. Second, antidepressants can help ease some people's pain and help them relax.

There are many kinds of painkillers, muscle relaxants, and anti-inflammatory drugs. Some you can buy over the counter and some you need have a doctor prescribe for you.

If you are already taking medications or supplements, be sure to tell your doctor and to watch out for drug interactions. The more medications you take, the higher your chances or developing negative side effects from drug interactions. Of course, you should always read the drug facts that come with each medication.

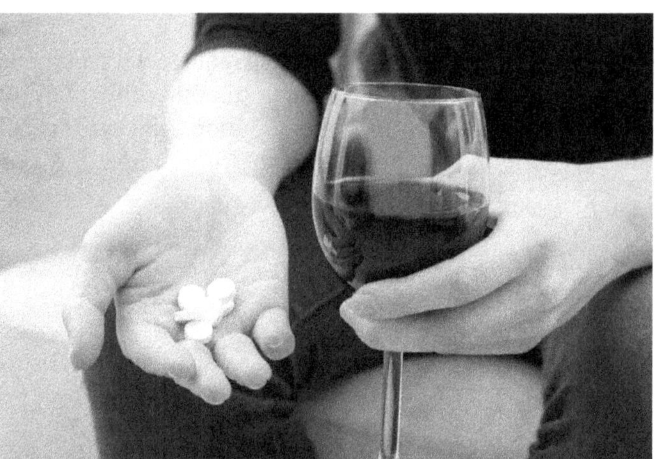

Do not take medications with alcohol.

Alcohol can change the effects of some medications. The change can seriously harm you.

Also, when you are taking painkillers, anti-inflammatories, or muscle relaxants, do not drive or do things that require a high degree of skill and concentration, where mistakes can cause serious injury to yourself or to others.

These drugs can relax you, slow down your reflexes, make your drowsy, and impair your judgement. Choose your activities carefully when you are taking these medications.

Medications are designed for short-term use. When you take them long-term, you have a higher chance of developing the side effects that they warn you about on the medication packaging.

Again, always read all the materials that come with any medication you take so that you can recognize if you are developing some of the side effects that they warn you about.

Besides increasing your chances of developing side effects when you take medications long-term, you will also increase your chances of developing an addiction to these drugs.

As I write this, many Americans are currently suffering from opioid addiction – turning their life and their family's life upside down. Hopefully, we can overcome our nation's opioid addiction problem.

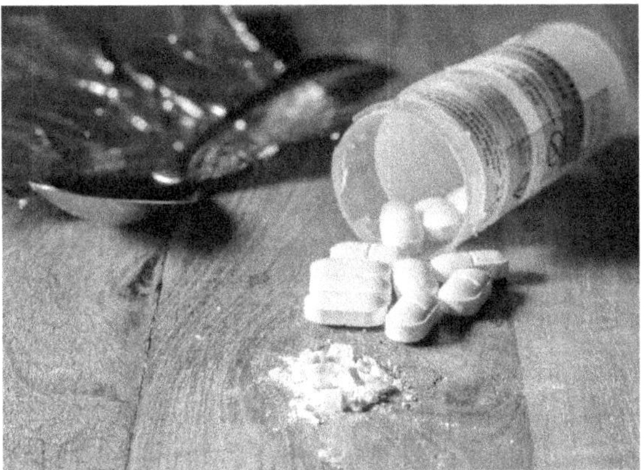

**In the meantime, the best thing you can do
is to not join the ranks of those addicted to opioids.**

If you are going to take addictive medications, work closely with your doctor to carefully plan your dosage and establish a plan to wean you off the medications that are designed for short-term use.

Dr. John Falkenroth, D.C.

19 SHOULD YOU GET
SPINAL INJECTIONS?

You might have heard of sciatica sufferers getting injections in their spine. These are typically epidural steroidal injections.

When you have sciatica, your body will create inflammation in any injured areas, which are usually around your herniated or bulged lumbar spinal discs and pinched or irritated sciatic nerve roots. Inflammation brings chemicals that irritate the tissues in the injured areas. This irritation causes pain.

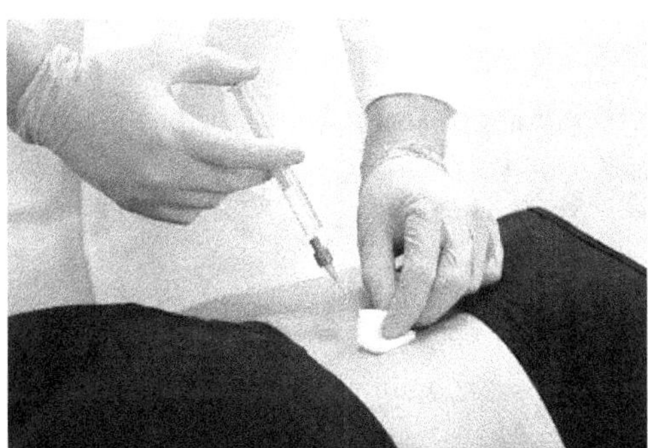

The main goal of the injection is to relieve pain.

The injected solution usually contains steroids, anesthetic, and saline solution. The steroid is designed to reduce and stop the inflammation. The local anesthetic will numb the pain. The saline solution will dilute the chemicals in the area causing pain. This is how spinal injections can help decrease sciatica pain.

If you are thinking of getting spinal injections for your sciatica, pick a doctor who has years of experience doing these injections. Doctors usually use imaging like fluoroscopy to help guide them in getting the needle placed in the proper spot.

A spinal steroid injection is usually safe and well tolerated by most patients. Unfortunately, like any medical procedure, spinal injections come with risks. For example, you can develop bleeding, nerve damage, or infection.

You might want to avoid spinal injections if you have bleeding problems or if you have a current infection in the site where the injection will happen or if you have an infection affecting your whole body.

Also, if you have a tumor or cancer causing your pain, doctors may not give you a spinal injection.

The spinal injection can also create a leakage of your spinal fluid causing you to feel a headache. To stop your headaches, a doctor needs to go back in and patch the leak.

Usually, this is done via a blood patch. In this process, they will draw blood from your vein and inject this blood into your epidural space. The hope is that the injected blood will plug the leak and stop your headaches.

After a spinal injection, you may retain fluids for a few days, so if you have kidney disease, diabetes or congestive heart failure, be sure to talk to your doctor to see if a spinal injection is safe for your condition.

Talk to your doctor if your pain gets worse after a spinal injection or if you develop a fever, a headache, or if you notice loss of function or loss of feeling in your arms, legs, bowel or bladder.

You should also keep in mind that you may not feel immediate pain relief after the injection. Usually, it takes a few days before patients notice a significant decrease in their pain.

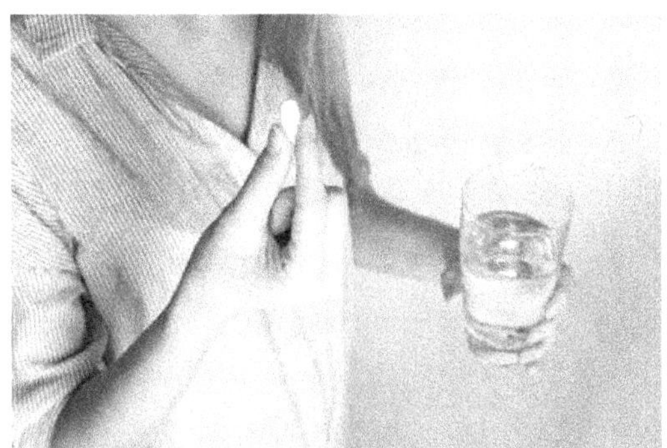

**This delayed pain relief is why some doctors recommend
that their patients continue to take painkillers
for a few days after a spinal injection.**

The pain relief that people get from spinal injections is usually temporary. This means that they need to keep going back to get more injections to relieve their pain. Unfortunately, chronic steroid use comes with a long list of undesirable side effects.

Since chronic use of steroids can harm you, doctors will usually not give their patients unlimited spinal steroidal injections.

Some doctors will only give their patients a maximum of 3 injections per year – or one every three to four months. Assuming your doctor did everything right and injected in the right spot, if you do not get pain relief after your first or second injection, then future spinal injections probably will not help you.

There is a time and place for spinal injections. For some patients, they may be beneficial. Talk to your doctor to see if spinal injections may be right for you.

20 IS SCIATICA SURGERY RIGHT FOR YOU?

If your sciatica gets much worse, and does not respond to conservative treatments, you may need sciatica surgery, which is back surgery.

Due to the invasive nature of surgery, medical researchers suggest that you should only consider sciatica surgery options if you meet the following criteria:

1. Severe leg pain for 6 weeks or longer
2. Sciatica not relieved by non-surgical sciatica treatment methods
3. Severe functional limitation
   OR
4. You are experiencing Cauda Equina Syndrome

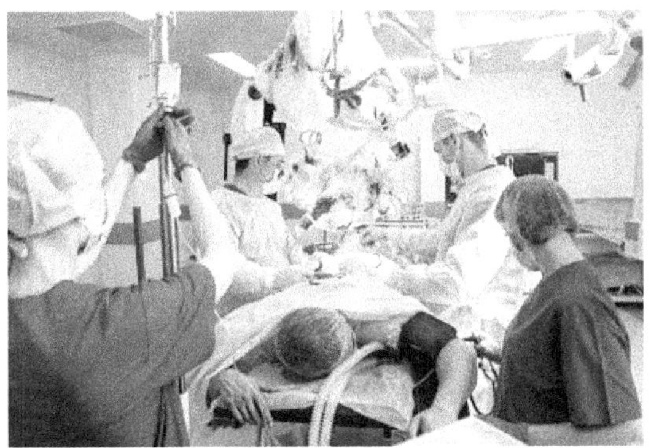

**Which back surgery you get
will depend on what is causing your sciatica.**

Since the most common cause of sciatica is disc herniations or disc bulges, most patients that undergo sciatica surgery get either a discectomy or a laminectomy.

If you have sciatica on one side, and it is caused by a herniated disc pinching on a sciatic nerve root, the sciatica surgery you will get will probably be a discectomy.

Discectomy involves surgically removing the part of the herniated disc that is pinching on the irritated sciatic nerve root.

Discectomies are done by cutting and opening your skin and connective tissue to allow access to the herniated disc. Usually, surgeons need to also cut or shave your vertebral bone (lumbar laminectomy or laminotomy) to see and to access your problematic herniated disc and nerve root.

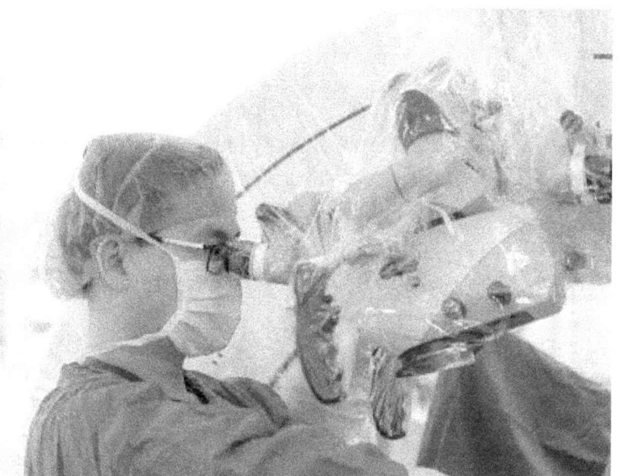

**Instead of cutting open your skin,
some back surgeons use a technique called
endoscopic discectomy or microdiscectomy.**

If you get a microdiscectomy, instead of cutting your skin and tissues, the surgeon will puncture your back with a tube that contains a camera or a microscope.

The surgeon will then use small surgical instruments inserted through the tube to cut off the herniated or bulged part of your disc.

Some back surgeons do not like to do endoscopic microdiscectomy, because they feel that their field of vision of the problematic area is limited. Some back surgeons prefer to do the traditional discectomies and therefore do not have as much experience in endoscopic microdiscectomy.

In addition to the discectomy or microdiscectomy, if you have other complicating conditions such as an epidural abscess, an epidural tumor, or Cauda Equina Syndrome adding to your nerve root compression, surgical treatment for these other conditions must also be performed.

As I mentioned earlier, in addition to the discectomy, a lumbar laminectomy or a laminotomy must be done in order to access the pinched nerve root and the herniated disc.

Although a disc herniation is the most common cause of sciatica, sciatica may also be caused by lumbar spinal stenosis. Spinal stenosis is narrowing of the spinal canal. This can pinch your spinal cord and spinal nerve roots.

There are many things that can cause spinal stenosis. For example, tumors, cysts, bleeding, fractures, thickening of spinal ligaments, bone spurs, and any other condition that can decrease your spinal canal area.

The most common cause of spinal stenosis is degeneration of the spine, as seen in aging, causing bone spurs and changes in spinal bone structure that results in narrowing of the spinal canal.

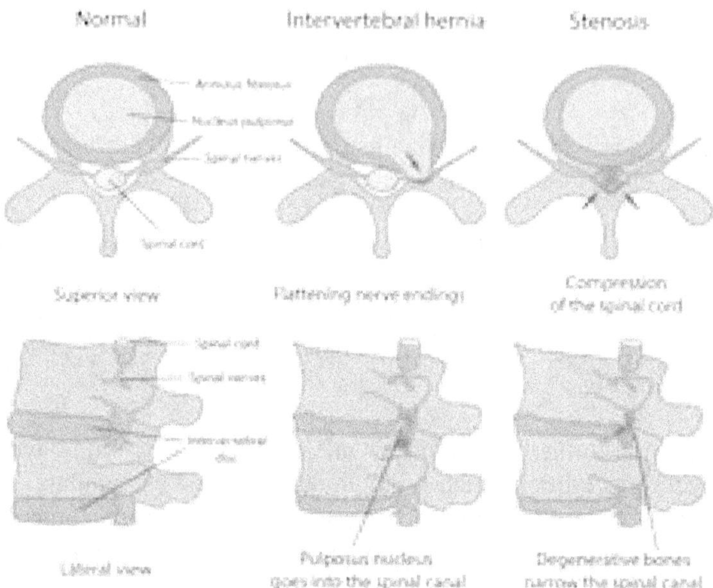

Disc herniations, spinal stenosis, and spinal disc degeneration can all narrow the spinal canal, often leading to sciatica.

If your sciatica is caused by spinal stenosis in your lumbar spine, the surgery of choice will probably be a lumbar laminotomy or a lumbar laminectomy.

Lumbar laminotomy surgically removes part of your affected lamina, which is a part of your vertebral bone. Lumbar laminectomy removes most of or all of the lamina that is causing your spinal stenosis.

Lumbar laminectomy is usually more invasive than the lumbar microdiscectomy that I talked about earlier.

If there is also a disc herniation complicating your lumbar spinal stenosis, a discectomy may also be done at the same time as the lumbar laminectomy, or each procedure can be done during two separate back surgeries.

If your back surgeon removes a significant amount of disc and bone material from your spine, your surgeon may need to fuse together the two vertebrae above and below your damaged disc and damaged spinal joints to keep those spinal segments stable. This additional, more invasive, surgical procedure is called spinal fusion.

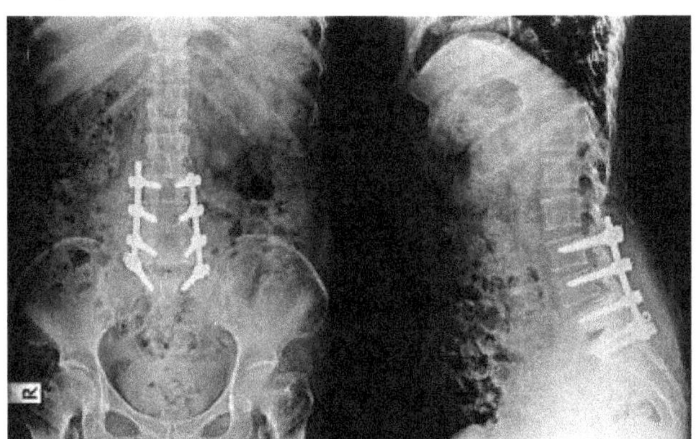

Spinal surgery usually involves placing hardware such as metal plates, screws, and cages into the spine.

Depending on your condition, some back surgeons recommend replacing specific damaged discs with artificial discs made of plastic or metal. This surgery is called artificial disc replacement.

If you want to see how lumbar laminectomy, lumbar discectomy, spinal fusion, and artificial disc replacement surgeries are done, you can search the internet for videos of these surgeries.

Keep in mind that for demonstration purposes, these surgical videos are usually shown as simplified 3-D spine models without all the other tissues and blood vessels in the area. The real surgeries are typically more complicated and messier.

Are You Healthy Enough
To Undergo Sciatica Surgery?

For all the sciatica surgery options mentioned above, you must be in good general health - especially if the sciatica surgery that you will be having is a lumbar laminectomy or spinal fusion.

Plus, in case your first surgery does not work, or if the back surgery makes your condition worse, you may need to have another back surgery done. This condition is referred to as Failed Back Surgery Syndrome

Multiple back surgeries require a healthy body for complete recovery - especially when the back surgeries are done within a close time frame.

This can be difficult for many sciatica sufferers, since many of them have become sedentary and out of shape due to their sciatica making it too difficult and painful to exercise and have a healthy active lifestyle.

Also, as with any form of surgery, post-surgical infection is always a risk. Your body must be very healthy to successfully combat post-surgical infections.

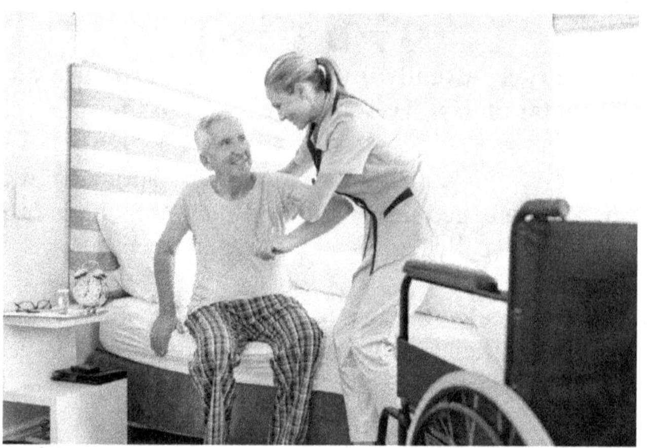

**You will need a lot of help
right after your back surgery.**

Depending on your specific condition, and which back surgery you get, sciatica surgery recovery can be painful and can take time. If you elect to have sciatica surgery, make sure you have someone who can help you during your recovery period.

After surgery, you will need to minimize bending, lifting, and twisting your back. Also, you will need to avoid driving, prolonged sitting, lifting heavy objects, and bending over. You may be limited to lifting things that only weigh 5 pounds or less.

After back surgery, you may need help with shopping, cooking, dressing, going to the bathroom, taking care of children and pets, cleaning, and doing your daily chores.

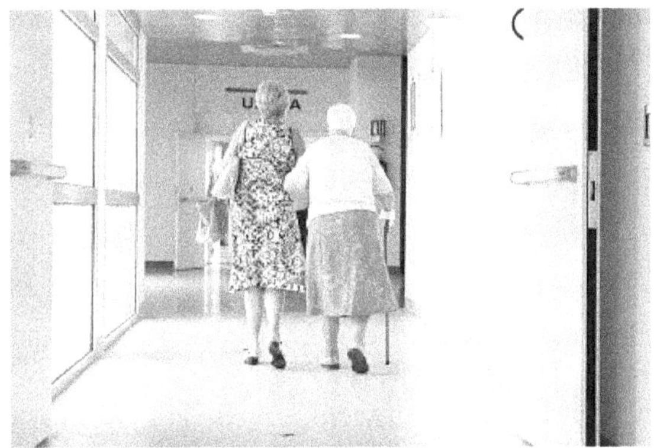

**You may also need help going to doctor's appointments
and physical therapy appointments.**

Think of all the activities of daily living that you currently do for yourself and for others and plan to have someone help you with those responsibilities - especially right after your surgery.

If you push yourself too hard and do not follow your surgeon's post-surgical care instructions, you may cause damage in the area where you had surgery and the problem that your surgeon worked on may come back.

Another thing to keep in mind when considering sciatica surgery is whether you are a "scar former."

As with any surgery that requires a cut or a penetration to your skin and connective tissue, a scar may form. This post-surgical scar tissue can complicate your recovery. Some people form more scar tissue or thicker scars after surgery than others.

These post-surgical scars can also pinch on your sciatica nerve roots and make your sciatica symptoms return or get worse. Surgery will usually leave a scar. Problematic scarring will depend on how much scar tissue your body develops.

In the beginning, post-surgical scarring may not be an issue, but as time goes by, some people continue to develop such severe post-surgical scarring that they must have another back surgery to remove the scar tissue. Then they must have another back surgery later to again remove the post-surgical scar tissues… and on and on.

This is a terrible cycle that you want to avoid.

What Are the Risks
Of Sciatica Surgery?

The risks depend on how invasive the procedure is and how severe your condition is. The best way for you to minimize your risks from surgery is to follow your surgeon's post-surgical instructions very closely. Otherwise, you may find yourself experiencing sprain or strain injuries and you may also re-herniate your surgically excised spinal disc.

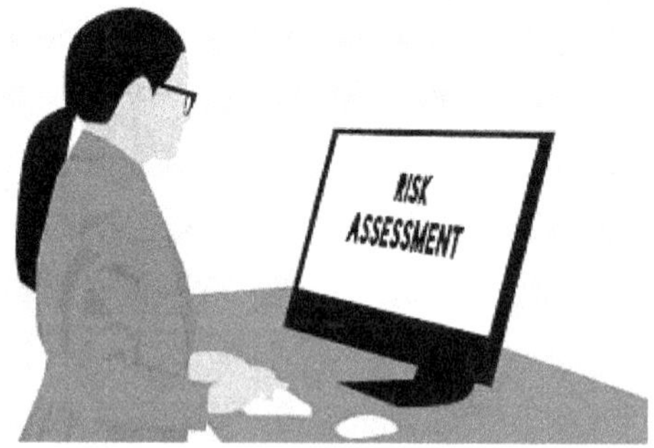

Surgeons and hospital staff do their best to minimize the risks, but like many surgeries, sciatica surgery come with risks.

Here is a *partial* list of the risks of sciatica surgery:

- Nerve root damage
- Dural tear causing cerebrospinal fluid leak
- Recurrent disc herniation
- Bladder or bowel incontinence
- Infection
- Bleeding

**How Much Does
Sciatica Surgery Cost?**

It depends on many factors. Like other medical procedures, it is hard to know exactly how much something costs. To learn more about sciatica surgery cost, call your medical insurance company and ask them how much sciatica surgery will cost you.

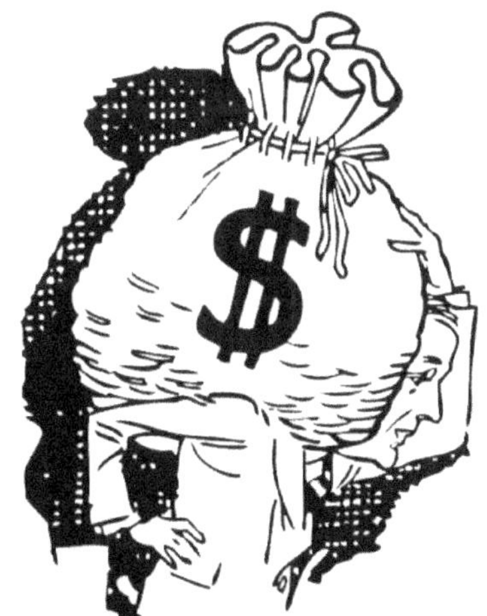

**It is best if you can plan ahead for payment of
your medical bills before going into surgery.**

Also, call your surgeon's office and the hospital where your sciatica surgery will be performed and ask them how much it will cost. Keep in mind that in many cases, you will be charged by the hospital for their facility use and staff cost. In addition, you will also be separately charged by each doctor – surgeon, anesthesiologist, and any other doctors who helped during your back surgery.

If your health insurance has different coverage for in-network providers and out-of-network providers, make sure the hospital and the doctors that will be taking part during your surgery are in-network with your insurance company.

Some insurance plans have no out-of-network benefits. If for example, one of the doctors that assisted during your back surgery is out of network with your insurance plan, you will need to pay that doctor's bill in full out of your own pocket without any participating provider fee discount.

Sometimes, you may not know ahead of time who the other doctors are who will be assisting your surgeon during your back surgery.

You will also most likely need physical therapy or rehabilitation treatments after your sciatica surgery and follow-up visits with your surgeon. Ask your insurance company about your coverage for these services as well.

It is best if you know the total cost of your sciatica surgery and post-surgical rehabilitation. You should have your payment arrangements in place before your surgery. This will allow you and your loved ones to focus on your recovery instead of focusing on paying your medical bills.

How Effective Is
Back Surgery for Sciatica?

Before even considering sciatica surgery, talk to your primary doctor and your back surgeon about the effectiveness of back surgery for your specific condition.

There is mixed and confusing research data on the effectiveness of back surgery. Some data shows that back surgery can bring sciatica relief.

When a surgeon operates on a healthy individual who suffers from sciatica, the problem is simple without other complicating conditions, and the surgeon has excellent skills, there is a greater likelihood of the sciatica surgery being successful.

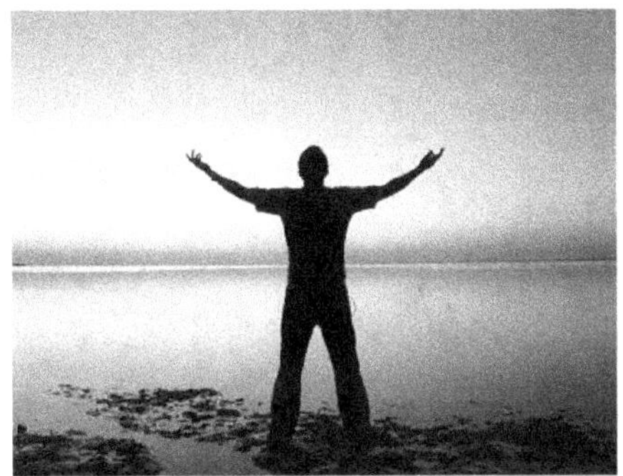

**No one wants to get back surgery,
but for some, it is a life changing procedure.**

Other data shows that even if surgery brings a patient relief from sciatica, the long-term outcome is about the same compared to if the patient chose to manage their sciatica using conservative, non-surgical treatment methods.

If your condition is still not severe, and you still have a choice of not getting sciatica surgery, keep looking for non-surgical sciatica solutions before committing to surgery.

What To Do If You Have No Choice
But To Undergo Back Surgery...

Unfortunately, there are times when your only option is back surgery. If this happens to you, do your best to make sure you are in top shape.

Because of your sciatica, you may be limited as far as exercising to get in shape. However, get proper hydration and nutrition to help you recover as quick as possible after your back surgery.

As I mentioned, put your financial plans in place to pay for your spinal surgery and rehabilitation. Line up the people who will help you during your surgery recovery.

Set up your house so that you can comfortably recover. Depending on your condition, you may have trouble going upstairs or accessing other areas of your house - especially during the first few days after your surgery.

Of course, you should pick a great back surgeon. There are many highly skilled back surgeons in this country.

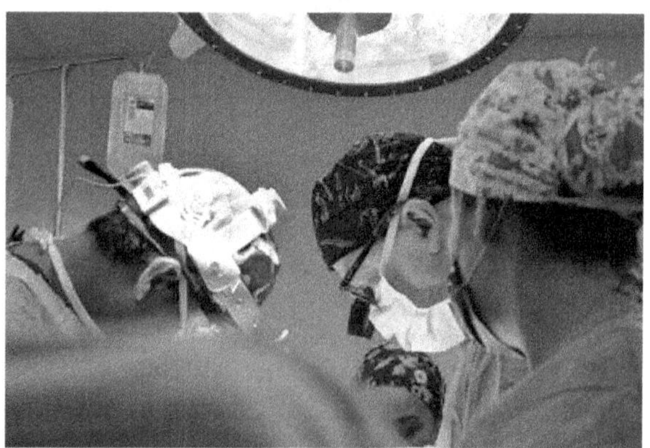

**Your fate depends on your back surgeon,
so do your research and pick a good one.**

One of the best things you can do to get confidence on your choice of back surgeon is to ask your surgeon how long they have been doing back surgeries and how many surgeries similar to the one they will perform on you have they done as the <u>lead</u> surgeon.

You should also hope for the best surgical outcome and a speedy recovery. Reassure yourself that your back surgeon will do their best and will do a great job, and that NOT everyone develops Failed Back Surgery Syndrome.

If you need to undergo back surgery, think of positive outcomes instead of the potential negative outcomes. In other words, HOPE FOR THE BEST AND STAY POSITIVE.

21 NON-SURGICAL SPINAL DECOMPRESSION THERAPY

If you do not want to get sciatica surgery, there are non-surgical treatment options that can help decompress your spine; relieve pressure on herniated, bulging, or degenerated discs; and relieve the pinching of your sciatic nerve roots.

Technological advances have given birth to many non-surgical therapies and treatments designed for people with back pain or sciatica who want to avoid back surgery.

One of these treatments is called Non-Surgical Spinal Decompression.

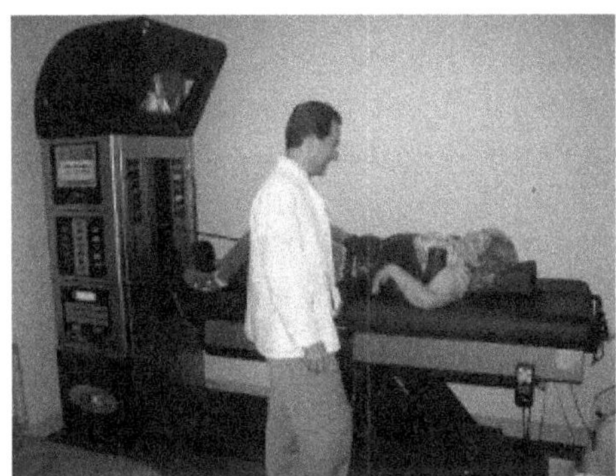

**This remarkable machine is one of the reasons
I have such a high success rate helping
patients with sciatica and low back pain.**

After over 20 years in practice, I have treated over 4,000 patients. Many of them had sciatica. I have been doing Non-Surgical Spinal Decompression with this machine for over 10 years. Most of my sciatica patients get fantastic results from this therapy.

It does not help EVERYONE with sciatica, but it may help you. Which one would you rather try - Non-Surgical Spinal Decompression or back surgery? If this treatment does not help you, you can still get back surgery. But, what if this treatment can save you from undergoing back surgery?

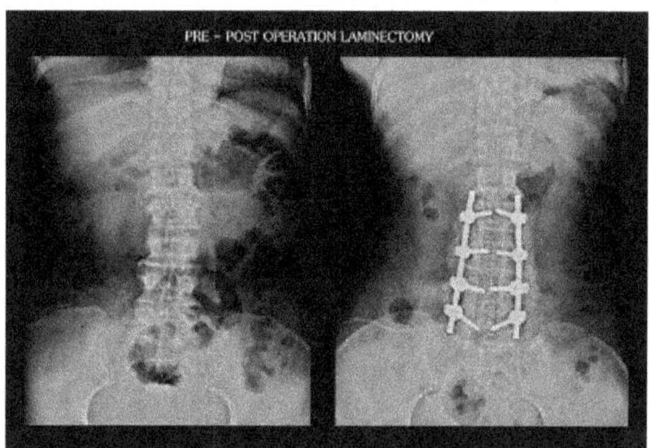

Here's a before and after x-rays of a patient who got surgery on their low back.

Some back surgeons recommend that their patients try Non-Surgical Spinal Decompression first before they operate on their backs. For many of their patients, this less invasive treatment lets their patients get rid of their pain without the need for back surgery.

When this treatment first came out, the success rate of this machine in treating low back pain impressed a lot of back pain doctors, including many back surgeons.

In addition to using the machine on my patients with low back pain, I use the machine on my sciatica patients. Most of my patients with sciatica get much needed relief after getting this treatment.

Being on this machine is very EASY and RELAXING.

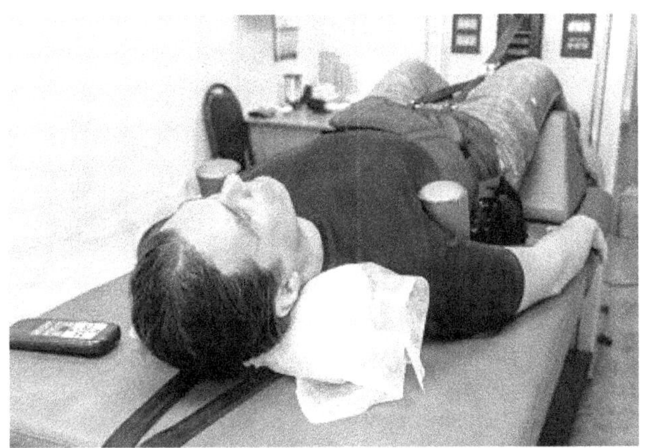

**Most of my patients that use this machine relax
and take a short nap during their session.**

For a lot of my sciatica patients, being on this machine is the only time when they have no leg pain or foot pain or numbness or tingling. Therefore, they are *finally* able to relax.

Many sciatica sufferers do not know about Non-Surgical Spinal Decompression. You should know that not all Non-Surgical Spinal Decompression treatments and therapies are of equal quality.

There are different machines out there and there are different doctors and technicians with varying degrees of training and experience that use these machines.

For best results, find a doctor in your area who has a track record of getting great results using Non-Surgical Spinal Decompression. If you happen to visit Santa Cruz County in California, where my clinic is located, call my clinic, or come by and see if your condition qualifies for treatment on this machine.

If you have tried other sciatica treatments and your sciatica is not better, you might want to consider this little-known sciatica treatment called Non-Surgical Spinal Decompression.

22 HOW AGING WREAKS HAVOC ON YOUR SPINE

Let's face it. We are all getting older. Unfortunately, as you age, the discs in your back and neck will break down and get weaker. This can cause you to develop bulging or degenerated discs.

Bulging discs can more easily become herniated discs than healthy, non-bulging discs. Having a herniated disc is like having a pebble in your spine that you cannot take out. This can lead to constant sharp pain, burning pain, numbness, pins and needles, or cramping that will not go away.

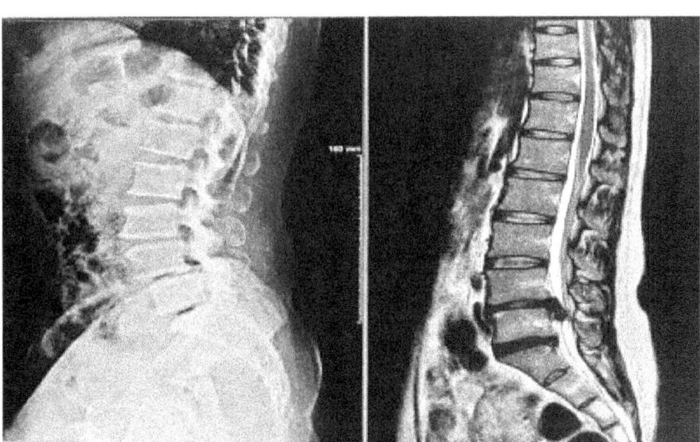

Here is an x-ray and an MRI of a degenerated lumbar spine. Notice the bone spurs and the herniated disc.

As you age, you will likely develop arthritis and bone spurs in your spine. Your body will try to stabilize your degenerating spine by making your spinal ligaments thicker. Your thicker ligaments can create spinal stenosis, choking not just your nerves, but also possibly pinching your spinal cord.

How will you know if your nerves are being pinched? You will feel back pain, neck pain, sciatica, tingling, numbness, or cramping in your neck, back, butt, arms, hands, legs, or feet. If your nerves get irritated and choked long enough, your nerves will start to develop permanent damage and degenerate. This will result in muscle loss in your affected arms, hands, legs, or feet.

You may not notice your lost muscle mass right away, but you will notice your muscles getting weaker. If the dying nerves are in your low back, you will notice the muscle weakness because you will be tripping, or your legs will feel weak - especially after long periods of standing or walking.

As your condition gets worse, you might develop a "foot drop," since you will have trouble lifting your foot off the ground. You might develop a limp when you walk. You might be forced to use a cane or a walker, not only to help you walk, but also to prevent you from falling and hurting yourself.

Your complete recovery depends on a lot of factors, but the top two things that determine whether you will recover fully are the severity of your nerve compression and how long the nerve has been compressed and left untreated.

Sometimes, the nerve can recover, and you can regain your normal function, but other times, the nerve can be permanently damaged, and your loss of function will be permanent.

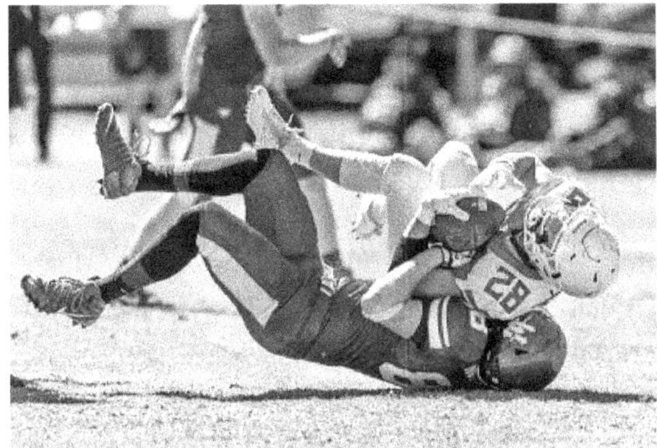

**Previous traumas or injuries to your spine
can speed up the aging of the injured areas.**

Aging of the spine is a slow process. BUT, if you've had a previous accident or trauma that affected your neck or back, this will speed up the wear and tear in the areas of your spine that got hurt - making these areas age faster. This is especially true if you have had multiple traumatic injuries.

You will most likely see bone spurs, bulging or herniated discs, and thicker ligaments much EARLIER in these injured spinal joints. Your body might even fuse two or more of your spinal bones together to try to stabilize your prematurely degenerated spinal joints.

Unfortunately, even without trauma, there are areas of your spine that tend to wear out more, because the nature of their anatomy makes them more likely to have more wear and tear. This is especially true at the base of your lower back and at the lower part of your neck.

You cannot stop aging and you cannot undo your past accidents, injuries, or traumas. You must do what you can to stop your aging spine from making you helpless, miserable, and disabled.

A little-known problem adds "fire" to the already existing mess that you may have in your back. When you hurt your back or neck, you can trigger the inflammatory process in the injured area. This means that you will get inflammation or swelling in the area. The fluid build-up from the swelling can irritate or pinch your nerves.

In addition to the excess fluids, you will also get inflammatory chemicals that are "toxic" to the bones, joints, and ligaments in your spine. These inflammatory chemicals can start a process called degenerative joint disease.

These chemical irritants can attack your discs, destroy your joint cartilage, and even ruin the protective tissues wrapped around your nerves. This may cause irreversible damage.

Uncontrolled inflammation in your spine is like degeneration on steroids. The sooner you can get your spine treated, the less permanent damage you will suffer from.

If we could see the damage and the decay happening in our spine, it would motivate many of us to take better care of our spine. Unfortunately, we only notice spinal problems when we feel pain, tingling, or numbness or when we see abnormalities on x-rays or MRIs of our spine.

In addition to creating pain and discomfort when your spinal nerves get pinched, these pinched nerves can also create dysfunction or disease in other parts of your body.

Besides working with your muscles, bones, ligaments, and joints, your spinal nerves also act as wires that relay messages between your brain and your body's organs.

Specific spinal nerves go to specific organs in your body. Irritated nerves in your spine can affect the quality of the communication between your brain and your affected organs. This can cause negative effects on the functioning of your organs.

How would you know if your organ function is compromised? The affected organ will not be functioning normally or optimally, therefore causing negative effects on your health. This can lead to various symptoms related to the affected organ.

VERTEBRAL LEVEL	NEVER ROOT	INNERVATION	POSSIBLE SYMPTOMS
C 1	C 1	Intracranial Blood Vessels • Eyes • Lacrimal Gland • Parotid Gland • Scalp • Base of Skull • Neck Muscles • Diaphragm	Headaches • Migraine Headaches • Dizziness • Sinus Problems • Allergies • Head Colds • Fatigue • Vision Problems • Runny Nose • Sore Throat • Stiff Neck • Cough • Croup
C 2	C 2		
C 3	C 3		
C 4	C 4		
C 5	C 5	• Neck Muscles • Shoulders • Elbows • Arms • Wrists • Hands • Fingers • Esophagus • Heart • Lungs • Chest	• Arm Pain • Hand and Finger Numbness or Tingling • Asthma • Heart Conditions • High Blood Pressure
C 6	C 6		
C 6	C 7		
C 7	C 8		
T 1	T 1	Arms • Esophagus • Heart • Lungs • Chest • Larynx • Trachea	Wrist,Hand and Finger Numbness or Pain • Middle Back Pain • Congestion • Difficulty • Breathing • Asthma • High Blood Pressure • Heart Conditions • Bronchitis • Pneumonia • Gallbladder Conditions • Jaundice • Liver Conditions • Stomach Problems • Ulcers • Gastritis • Kidney Problems
T 2	T 2		
T 3	T 3		
T 4	T 4		
T 5	T 5	Gallbladder • Liver • Diaphragm • Stomach • Pancreas • Spleen • Kidneys • Small Intestine • Appendix • Adrenals	
T 6	T 6		
T 7	T 7		
T 8	T 8		
T 9	T 9		
T 10	T 10		
T 11	T 11	Small Intestines • Colon • Uterus	
T 12	T 12	Uterus • Colon • Buttocks	
L 1	L 1	Large Intestines • Buttocks • Groin • Reproductive Organs • Colon • Thighs • Knees • Legs • Feet	Constipation • Colitis • Diarrhea • Gas Pain • Irritable Bowel • Bladder Problems • Menstrual Problems • Low Back Pain • Pain or Numbness in Legs
L 2	L 2		
L 3	L 3		
L 4	L 4		
L 5	L 5		
	SACRAL	Buttocks • Reproductive Organs • Bladder • Prostate Gland • Legs • Ankles • Feet • Toes	Constipation • Diarrhea • Bladder Problems • Menstrual Problems • Lower Back Pain • Pain or Numbness in Legs

**A spinal nerve chart shows possible symptoms
of nerve irritation or pinching.**

If you look at a spinal nerve chart, you will discover that certain spinal nerves go to certain organs. You can see if the areas where you have back pain or neck pain correlate to other symptoms that you are having.

If there is a correlation, an irritated spinal nerve may be contributing to your symptoms or other health challenges.

Sometimes a chiropractic spinal adjustment alone can relieve your nerve irritation - especially if you get treated soon after you develop spinal joint misalignment or spinal joint motion problems.

23 WHAT YOU CAN DO TO SLOW DOWN THE AGING OF YOUR SPINE

Fortunately, there are still things that can be done to help slow the wear and tear process of your spine.

First, you need to STOP doing damage to your spine. Second, you need to give your spine the proper nutrition and environment to heal and to thrive in. Third, you need to do stretching and strengthening exercises of your spinal muscles and ligaments and core musculature. Refer to earlier chapters to remember how to do these.

It is also important to keep each joint of your spine moving. This will help prevent pre-mature aging of your spine. One of the best ways to keep each joint of your spine moving is to go to a skilled chiropractor on a regular basis and have them check for and correct any stuck or misaligned joints in your spine.

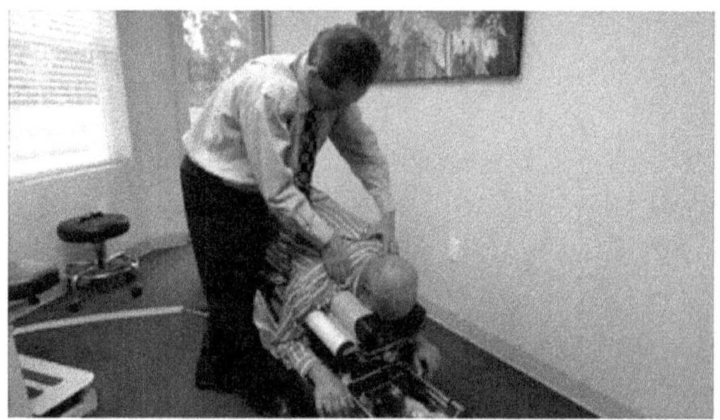

**A chiropractic treatment is
called an adjustment.**

One of the reasons why you feel better after a chiropractic adjustment is because you regain normal movement in an area of your spine that has been stuck or misaligned.

Just like other joints, lack of movement in your spinal joints makes them stiff, undernourished, dehydrated, and prone to decay or degeneration – problems that can speed aging of your spine and your body.

Chiropractic adjustments also help keep your spinal bones aligned and not abnormally rubbing on other parts. Thus, proper spinal alignment decreases the wear and tear on your spine. A well-aligned spine stays healthy longer, just like a well-aligned tire lasts longer.

If getting your spine cracked or twisted scares you, find a chiropractor that can adjust your spine with an instrument or with another method of gentle treatment. There are many ways to get your spine adjusted. Find the one that works best for you.

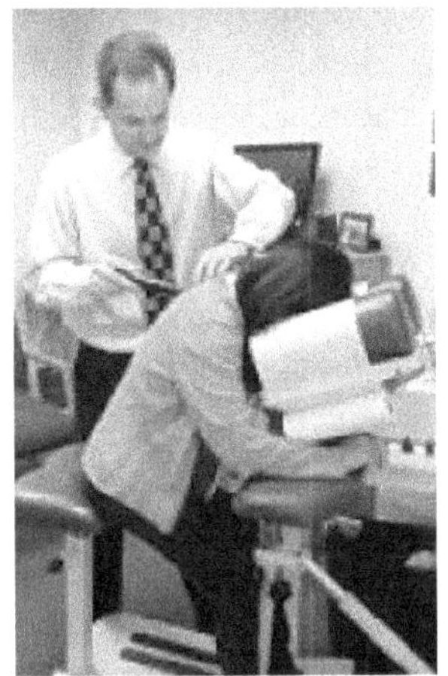

**A computer-guided adjusting instrument is one of the
tools I use to adjust my patients who do not like their
spines to be cracked, popped, or twisted.**

If you have bulging discs, herniated discs, or disc degeneration
complicating your situation, you may need more than a spinal
adjustment. You may also need other treatments such as Non-Surgical
Spinal Decompression therapy.

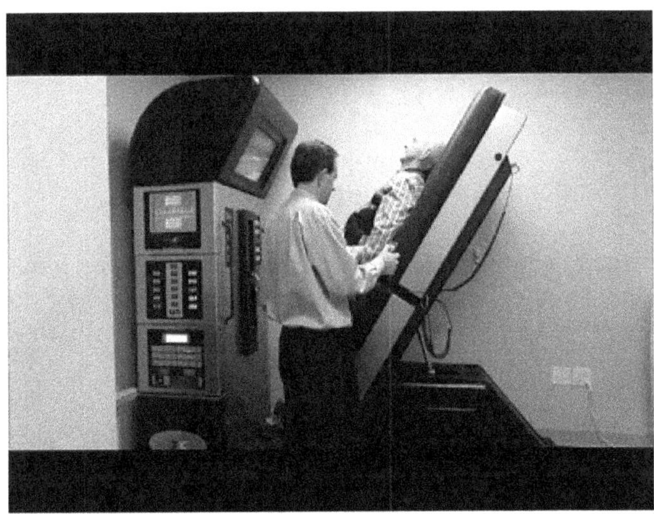

**I use Non-Surgical Spinal Decompression to
help patients with back pain and sciatica.**

My job is to help my patients get relief of their back pain, sciatica symptoms, or neck pain. There is also a MORE important part of my job, which is to help my patients AVOID losing their ability to do what they need to do in their lives.

If you are like most of my patients, you probably need to work to make a living - doing things that require a healthy spine. It is my responsibility to you and your family that I help you with your sciatica, so that you can do your job and provide for yourself and for your family.

You may be retired and still living in your own house. I want you to be able to continue to function well enough so that you can continue to live independently, and not burden your family and friends with taking care of you.

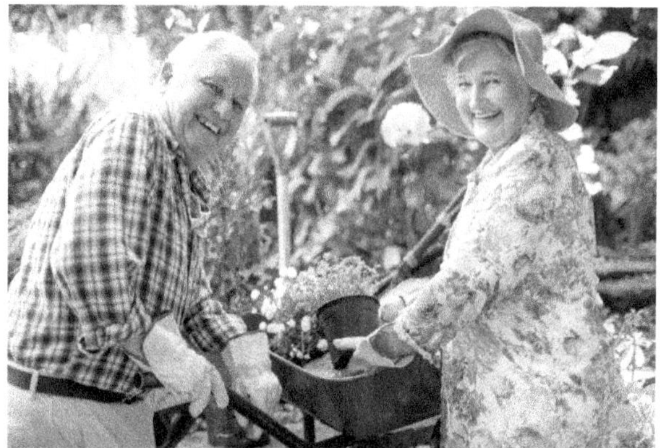

**One of the greatest joys in life is
living independently in our later years.**

I want you to enjoy that privilege of independent living for as long as you can. What you do with your spine today determines how your spine will feel later in life – and can affect how well you can take care of yourself as you get older.

You may have hobbies or other activities that you love doing that require a healthy spine such as traveling, playing sports, hiking, gardening, and playing with your kids and grandkids. I want you to be able to continue with your active lifestyle and not have to give up what you love doing.

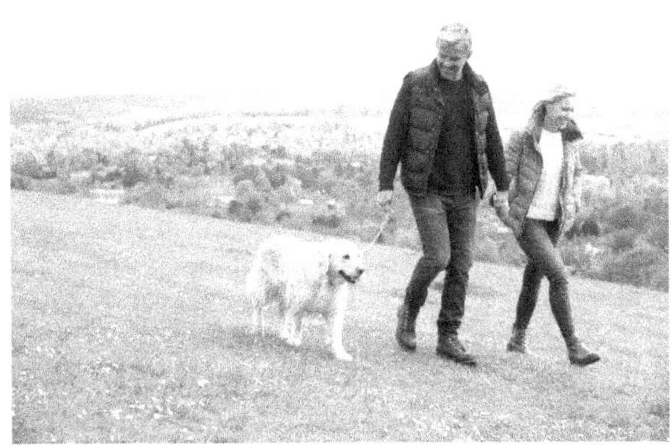

After all, life is about doing what you love with the people you love.

After over 20 years of treating thousands of patients with back pain and sciatica, I strongly encourage you to find a chiropractor to monitor and adjust your spine on a regular basis before you develop serious spinal problems that can cause you pain and suffering and can inconvenience you and your family.

Thank you for taking the time to read this book. I hope it helped you understand your sciatica better. I hope it gave you useful strategies to help relieve your sciatica symptoms.

I also hope that reading this book will motivate you to take great care of your spine so that you can avoid future pain, disability, suffering, and dependence on others.

Encourage your friends and family to take care of their spine or they may end up with a debilitating back problem or sciatica.

Whatever next steps you take with your sciatica, I wish you the best. If you are ever in Santa Cruz County in California, and you would like my help with your sciatica, I would be honored to work with you and help you.

If you want more information on sciatica treatments and other things that can help you relieve your sciatica symptoms, please visit our websites at **sciaticaacademy.com** and **repairmyback.com**.

ABOUT THE AUTHOR

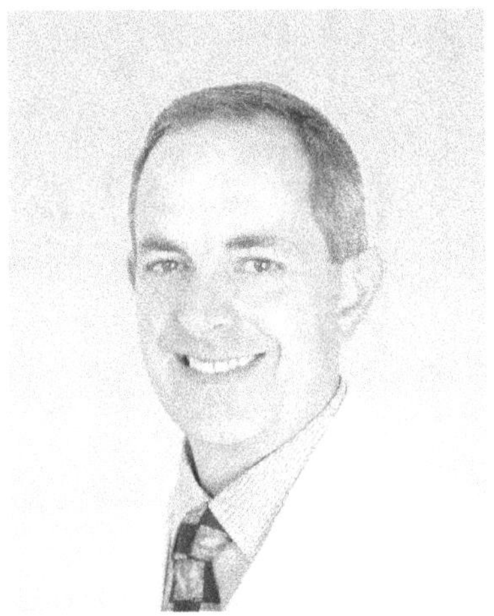

Dr. John Falkenroth, D.C. is the Clinic Director at the Back Pain and Sciatica Clinic in Soquel, California, USA. After over 20 years in practice, Dr. Falkenroth has helped over 4,000 patients - many of them who were suffering from sciatica.

Prior to receiving his doctorate at chiropractic college, Dr. Falkenroth attended the University of California at Davis, where he earned a Bachelor of Science Degree in Physiology in 1994.

While studying human physiology at the University of California at Davis, Dr. Falkenroth learned how irritation or impingement of the spinal nerve roots as they exit the spine can negatively affect a person's health.

With this realization, Dr. Falkenroth decided to help others by becoming an expert in treating back pain, neck pain and sciatica.

To complement his physiology background from UC Davis, Dr. Falkenroth decided to go to Davenport, Iowa, USA to attend the 120+ year old top-rated chiropractic college in the world – Palmer College of Chiropractic – where he graduated *summa cum laude* in 1998.

Go to **www.repairmyback.com** and **www.sciaticaacademy.com** for more sciatica relief tips.